Unlocked

RELEASE YOUR PEAK POTENTIAL AND REBUILD A BODY
THAT'S FUTURE-PROOF

Richard Gliddon, DC

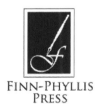

FINN-PHYLLIS
PRESS

Unlocked / Richard Gliddon - 1st ed.

ISBN 978-1-7330337-4-9 (eBook)

ISBN 978-1-7330337-5-6 (pbk)

Cover design by Jetlaunch.net

Edited by Elizabeth Lyons

http://www.spinecentral.co.uk

Contents

Legal Disclaimer

This book is not intended as a substitute for the medical advice of a physician. The reader should regularly consult a physician in matters relating to his/her health, and particularly with respect to any symptoms that may require diagnosis or medical attention.

Foreword

Many things can be said about Advanced BioStructural Correction™, but they can be summed up by saying that practitioners can return your body to health beyond what you can currently imagine. For many, the most typical question at the beginning of treatment is, "Remember those things you used to be able to do that you no longer can?" After they answer, the practitioner states, "Within a few months, and without even thinking about it, you will find yourself doing many of them again with no special effort or pain. In the long term, you will find your body working so well that you will be as active as you want to be, doing all your desired activities, without having any attention on your body at all."

In *Unlocked*, Richard Gliddon explains how and why you will be able to simply live your life and do whatever you want to do with no attention on your body. It will just work.

—*Dr. Jesse Jutkowitz, Founder of Advanced BioStructural Correction™*

Introduction

As I lay flat on the ice, it felt as if time had stopped. A high-pitched ringing sound pierced through my head as I desperately gasped for breath. No matter how hard I tried, I could not draw in a single drop of air. It was as though my throat had been sealed shut. I continued gasping for what seemed like an eternity, and as I grew increasingly desperate, a deflating sense of relief flowed through me as I realised, in a moment of clarity, that I could still move my toes.

Just moments before, I was snowboarding down the slope towards the same half-pipe I had enjoyed riding three times earlier that morning. Only this time, with an air of confidence, I never slowed down. I pointed my board straight for the wall, tucked in deep, hit it at full speed, and launched myself well clear of the top. What I hadn't anticipated was that, thanks to a full morning of strong sunshine and plenty of use, the wall of the half-pipe had become eroded and undercut. Due to its newly formed crescent shape, I was not only launched skywards but also away from the wall. Instead of simply turning and landing on the smooth incline, I fell a long way down onto hard, unyielding ice. I landed feet-first, but my board skidded out from underneath me, and as my backside bit the deck I was forcefully compressed in half, creating an explosion of bones.

While I didn't know it at the time, the two spinal compression fractures created in that moment set off a chain of events that would forever change the way I approached my life's work. They were to become my single greatest teacher. Frustratingly, painfully, and faithfully they guided me on a journey of discovery that would turn upside down nearly everything I thought to be true about spinal health, transforming the lives of thousands of people in the process.

Up until that moment, I considered myself to be one of the very best in the business of structural health (focusing on everything related to bones, joints, muscles, and nerves). I had built a large, busy chiropractic practice and helped thousands of people find relief from their various aches, pains, injuries, and health problems. My desire to be among the best combined with my innate passion for all things health-related led me on a seemingly never-ending quest to learn as much as I could. I studied far and wide, knew many different chiropractic techniques in depth, and had accumulated an extensive knowledge about the nutritional, mental, emotional, and lifestyle aspects of healing. It worked. My team and I were able to help the majority of patients who came through our doors. I loved my work, and never tired of it. The problem was, it didn't work *for me* when I desperately needed it to.

The four years following my snowboarding accident increasingly became overshadowed by back pain and stiffness. My business continued to grow, but I was less and less able to handle the workload. After a day of adjusting patients, I would sit on the train home wanting to crawl out of my skin to escape the feeling of being "all seized up." There was no escaping the deep tension and relentless ache. Most evenings when I got home, I'd lie flat on the floor for an hour or more just to get some relief. The thought of doing it all again the next day began to weigh heavily on my mind, and I was forced to reconsider what the future may bring. Enjoyment of the physical side of life had been all but removed from my life—somewhat ironically as a result of the very problem I prided myself on helping others solve.

The worst part was the way it affected my energy and my mood. Everyone knows that chronic pain is a real buzzkill, but there is much more going on beneath the surface of the pain. The altered alignment, movement, and neurology of spinal injuries can "right care" at the time. A scenario I saw more than once was one wherein the same lower-back adjustment that had "fixed" thousands of people before ended up aggravating the complaint, or in some cases, resolved the back pain but led to a mysterious shoulder pain, headache, or foot pain that wasn't there before. When I sat down and thought about these facts clearly, I could come to only one conclusion: my treatment methods were incomplete, and there was a deeper level of understanding that was missing. The new science of ABC™ plugged all of those holes.

After twelve years in clinical practice, I am more convinced than ever that the single most overlooked area in healthcare is the body's structure. Your body is essentially a highly complicated machine, and structural health is concerned with the alignment and mechanical function of all of your joints, bones, ligaments, tendons, fascia, and nerves working together as a single functioning system. When this system works correctly, you get to experience your life unrestricted and faithfully supported by a robust frame. This system not only helps you to get on with being productive and enjoying your life, it also has direct implications upon your health. Every organ and every system is directly and intricately linked to your mechanical function. Your alignment really does matter.

Most people are completely unaware of how or why their body begins to betray them. When it does, they spend lots of time, energy, and money seeking treatment, which all too commonly does not provide the level of sustained relief they are seeking. For this reason, there is a predictable decline in structural health seen throughout the Western world as people age. This is most commonly exposed as a progressively forwards-stooped posture. Just take a look around at the average person over age fifty (although problems can begin a lot sooner, even in early childhood) and you will see that most people are literally stuck forwards. That degenerative postural decline is optional; it's not a required outcome for a modern-day human being.

Over the years, I have noticed that the most pressing question on the minds of new patients is, "Why does my body hurt, and how did it get to be like this?" The next most common question is, "How can we fix it?" To answer those questions based on conventional understanding that exists in the field of healthcare is quite a challenge. It requires an entire book, in fact, to do it justice. This is why Chapter 1 addresses the flaw in the fundamental thinking that drives modern healthcare. It is only when you understand the lens through which conventional healthcare views your body that you can begin to see the real issues clearly—as well as the solutions that will take you where you want to go. The additional chapters will take you on a journey of learning how your body operates under the physical laws of the universe, how and why the human machine breaks down, and how to restore it back to good working order.

If you are currently looking for answers in your own health, you probably understand firsthand how hard it can be to know which way to turn. The wider perspective of alternative and complementary therapies have quite a range of opinions to sway you, from the fully converted *It transformed my life* to the rigidly ambivalent *There's no high-quality evidence to support its use, therefore it doesn't work* to the vehemently opposed *It's potentially dangerous and can delay medical treatment so don't go near it.*

These attitudes, together with the complicated reality that healthcare is a soft science, not a hard science—meaning that not all treatments work for all bodies—can make it really tough to know which way to turn.

I am hyper-aware of these important issues, having experienced the full range of patient outcomes myself, as both a practitioner and a patient. Mentally wrestling with these issues was one of my driving motivations to find better solutions.

The important difference that I bring to this complex and noisy landscape is that I have practiced this pioneering new approach to structural healthcare for five full years. During that time, I have seen it deliver consistently amazing results for bodies of all shapes, sizes, genders, and ages with a level of predictability that is simply unrivaled. I have seen these results through the experienced and hyper-critical eye of the seven previous years I spent using a highly specific and detailed—albeit traditional—approach to chiropractic care. Much of the time, I was attempting to disprove the claims that Advanced BioStructural Correction founder, Dr. Jesse Jutkowitz, made. I figured that the best way to find out if the method was all it was cracked up to be was to go all-in and master it. Only then would I have a direct comparison and the certainty I sought for our patients. I wanted to accept based upon results, not simply theory, that a science of rebuilding bodies really did exist.

ABC™ is an applied science of biomechanics that combines some incredible new discoveries about how bodies work that have quite simply been overlooked in last hundred years or so. Results are demonstrable in the here and now. You don't have to wait for healing to occur in order to notice firsthand, or observe as an outsider, the body improving mechanically right before your eyes. The principles embodied in the ABC™ method of care are so fundamental to the way your body was designed to work that, if ignored, your results will become more unpredictable and inconsistent. Once you understand these principles and how they apply to your body, you will grasp on a much deeper level why so much complexity, confusion, and contradiction exists in the first place. And, it is really important that you learn and apply these principles because we are facing something of a healthcare crisis in the modern age.

THE HEALTHCARE CRISIS

As a species, we are getting sicker and sicker with each year that passes. Despite incredible advances in medical technology and more money than ever being spent on doctors and hospitals, in the area of structural healthcare alone, there are currently an estimated 1.6 billion people around the world suffering from chronic pain conditions. That's a hefty percentage of the world's population. The consequences of this in terms of lost productivity and reduced quality of life are huge. When you consider that people with pain are far less likely to move enough, let alone exercise, you can appreciate just how important an issue this is in the context of all the chronic health conditions that plague modern humans the world over.

We are living in a smartphone-laden, hyper-connected era, wherein the majority of people are sat, looking down at a TV, laptop, desktop computer, or mobile phone for long stretches of time. These modern habits wreak havoc on the human frame, trapping people into a cycle of postural decline and sedentarism. We simply do not move our bodies as if our lives depended upon it, and yet they absolutely do.

Good movement patterns and structural health (often thought of as "good posture") are among the most basic fundamentals of good health, and they are becoming increasingly rare qualities in the progressively more stationary human race. There is a price to pay for this unfortunate decline in the human condition: lost function. Everything from emotions to blood pressure, physical comfort, depth and ease of breathing, cognitive abilities, and athletic ability is directly related to your posture and ability to move easily and often throughout your day.

The fortunate side to this tale of woe is that the science and methodology to reverse this trend now exists. I did not make this important discovery, but I have taken full advantage of it, not only for my own healing but also to help thousands of people once again enjoy their bodies and regain years (if not decades) of lost function.

As a driven, high-performance individual, it's critical that you understand why body structure is so incredibly important to living a long and high-impact life that allows you to reach your highest potential while avoiding unnecessary health decline and injury. Through this book, my goal is to teach you this new biomechanical science of how your human machine works, why it goes wrong, and what you can do to rebuild and heal it.

I will frequently use the term "mechanism" because it literally references the way your body works. The body is a machine, and it works through the laws of physics. People move in three-dimensional space under the influence of gravity, and their bodies are machines with predictable mechanical ways. If you've ever seen the inside of a watch, you know that it's series of spinning cogs. That's the mechanism inside that machine. That particular machine doesn't work against gravity, but it has a lot of moving parts, just as the human body does. When you twist your neck, the force imparts changes throughout your entire body. People think that they can simply stretch out tight muscles and strengthen weak ones in order to fix their pain and poor posture, but what they're actually doing with this approach is neglecting to correct the mechanical problems that lead to the symptoms in the first place. The cogs were out of alignment, and no amount of tinkering with the hands will restore normal mechanical function to that machine. You have got to get to the root cause.

This isn't a belief system. It's the applied science of biomechanics. That fact makes it highly predictable and repeatable for treating the full spectrum of structural problems, which is in stark contrast to other treatment options that neglect to address the primary mechanical faults. Most practitioners are directly treating downstream effects, *thinking* that they are the cause, yet they aren't getting consistent, predictable results from their treatment. And, even when they do get results, they're only measuring them against the body parts that feel "looser" or have a reduction in pain. But what's happened to the way that the whole human machine works?

What happened to the overall alignment and posture? When I first learned ABC™, I was blown away by the poor posture that even my "best" clients had, despite the fact that, symptomatically, they were better.

If you have picked up this book, it's likely that you are searching for answers that address the deeper cause. You're looking for real results and want to get your younger, pain-free, fully functional body back. Perhaps you have back pain, neck pain, headaches, or a sporting injury that led you to seek help. Or, maybe you are aware of a gradual tightness, stooping forwards, and loss of performance that has crept up on you over the years. Regardless of whether you're trying to solve a problem or find a higher level of health, this book will help you understand the essential path to natural healing.

It will also help you navigate the highly complex world of complementary and alternative health. How do you know which practitioner is best for you, or which treatment process you should follow? There are many options to choose from, from chiropractic to osteopathy, physiotherapy, massage, and beyond. I will show you that, while all of these professions treat the same problems and share common approaches, the majority of practitioners who employ them are still using traditional methods, which fail to improve the body structure as a whole. Why? Because they fail to address the real underlying reason one's body mechanics have gone awry in the first place.

Structural correction has healed my own body to a point beyond which I ever thought possible. I have regained a level of athleticism that I thought was reserved for the genetically gifted, and my physical body has become my greatest asset in my search for personal growth and a life of adventure. Imagine being able to say goodbye to your aches, pains, and stiffness for good. Imagine waking up in the morning feeling loose and energised because you slept soundly through the night. Imagine getting to the end of the day, still feeling energised and alert, yet able to relax at will. Imagine being able to breathe easily and deeply, stand up tall without effort, and reach that next level of performance in your sports or hobbies. Imagine being able to swim, run, cycle, lift weights, or play tennis without your body tightening up and needing several days to recover. And most importantly, imagine being able to maintain this high level of function well into your old age.

Your chosen sport, profession, age, and—to some degree—physical disability or body structure issue, don't matter. With implementation of the methodology and tools that I teach in this book, you too can have your human machine restored to its highest performing state. Remember this important distinction: feeling your best, having high energy, sleeping well, feeling grateful, moving with ease, being pain-free, thinking clearly, and being athletic and robust are all side effects of good health. They are the natural set point for human beings whose bodies are working correctly. Disease, symptoms, and injuries simply reflect an absence of health, and even more accurately in this context, are a sign of an upstream lifestyle error that has created a mechanical problem and forced your body to adapt in order to survive.

Those years spent figuring out my own pain led me to discover the unflappable biomechanical science of structural correction. With the use of this method, I have been able to help patients get their bodies back and also gain the understanding of why doing this sort of work even matters. It goes beyond the desire to be pain free. The truth is, beneath it all, one of the most precious assets we can have in life is a healthy and robust body. Structural correction delivers what I firmly believe to be the greatest product in existence: structural health. What could be more exciting and more beneficial than restoring your human machine back to its best, and profiting from the cascading benefits that this brings to all areas of your life?

Whether you are suffering a great deal or simply know that your body isn't firing on all cylinders, I'm here to tell you that you can get your body back. Yet it goes even beyond that because many people are blissfully unaware of the slow, insidious loss of function that precedes the main problem. As humans, we are very good at adapting to new normals. We assume that stiffness, niggles, aches, fatigue, and grumpiness are to be expected. We grow indifferent to their burden, blind to the prison walls that have closed in around us, and unaware of the reduced capacity we have to explore, experience, and adapt to all that life brings. Curiously, most people stand to gain what they've long since forgotten they once had. The surprise recapturing of lost function is arguably the most rewarding part of the entire journey.

Structural correction is a methodology that can systematically, predictably, and consistently unlock your body from the burden of its mechanical problems, allowing you to go about life unrestricted. That is, after all, what your body was designed to do—quietly support all that you do as the faithful, selfless servant through which you accomplish great things.

WHAT THIS BOOK IS ALL ABOUT

A few words on what to expect in this book. This is not a typical self-help book on posture. There will be no long list of exercises on how to *self*-correct your body for the simple reason that you cannot stretch and strengthen your way to ideal alignment—not when you get down to the fundamentals of how the body actually works. Many have tried, and all approaches are superficial and of limited help, producing results that are transient at best. The funny thing is, so many people struggle with change. Yet change is easy. You can change pretty much anything in the instant you decide to. Your posture, for example, can be improved in an instant by tucking your pelvis and lifting your chest. The trouble with change, however, is that it is temporary. What you really need is transformation, and that can only come from making deep shifts to the fundamentals that drive the results you seek. What this book describes is the transformative process that fundamentally corrects the key issues that cause body pain, posture, and performance problems. It is journey of unlocking the natural strength and ideal alignment that is integral to the human design. It is about rediscovering the freedom of movement and living unrestricted, fully supported by your body. Getting to this level of result requires a fundamental shift in how you view your body.

I have three goals for this book. The first is to arm you with knowledge of how your skeletal frame works in the physical world, and why it goes wrong. This understanding is the single most important piece of the puzzle because from that point forward, you will know the best path to take in order to properly look after your body. It will become much easier to navigate the maze that is structural health care and all of the confusion and frustrations that surround the reasons why your body is no longer working at its best. You will understand why different practitioners give you different diagnoses for the same problems, and you will have clear understanding and direction around what needs to be done to get your body back. This is the foundation-level work that is so often missing in conventional teaching.

My second goal is to show you why your alignment matters. Many of us are blissfully unaware of the way that alignment intertwines and interacts with just about every aspect of our physical and mental health. You cannot help but be awestruck and appreciative for the body you have when you understand just how much it does for you.

My final goal is to teach you how to avoid the common and classic lifestyle mistakes that cause the majority of the structural health problems that plague humanity today. Outside of freak accidents, most of your aches, pains, and injuries are caused by a failure to appreciate that your body is a precision machine, and as such, it is subject to the same mechanical laws of physics as is the rest of the universe. Put too much pressure on it in ways that exceed its intended design, and there is an inevitable price to pay. Fortunately, most people get it wrong through simple life habits that are easy to correct. It is a winnable game, and a few simple tweaks to the way you go about sitting, sleeping, standing, and sports can make an exceptional difference to your quality of life as well as give you a very fair advantage in the game of life.

Let's begin.

CHAPTER 1

In Order to Build Tall, You Must Dig Deep

"If you have built castles in the air, your work need not be lost; that is where they should be. Now put foundations under them."

—*Henry David Thoreau*

Eighteen months ago, I walked down a street in London called the Upper Richmond Road. They had recently demolished multiple old office buildings and walled them off as building sites. That was the way things remained for much of the next year. I could just barely see over the fences to make out the tops of the diggers, cranes, and workers' porter cabins.

Day after day, I'd walk past these sites and hear a general buzz of activity from the jackhammers, diggers, and workers, but there was no visible sign that anything productive was happening. This apparent lack of progress continued for almost a year. And then, one day, it was possible to the see the first floors beginning to be completed. A month later, the external eight-story shell of the buildings was complete. These monsters literally sprang up, seemingly out of nowhere, up and down the street. No fewer than six eight-story blocks of flats shot up in a matter of days.

During the months when nothing appeared to be progressing, guess what they were doing? From the outside, it would appear not much. Yet, behind those walls, they were methodically and tirelessly digging the foundation, securing a stable platform upon which to build. This is arguably the most important phase of development when building structures because, unless the foundation is rock solid, there is no chance of supporting a skyscraper.

Consider for a moment the idea that your body is like a building. The foundation and support beams are your skeleton, the walls are your muscles, the various rooms are your organs, the smart electrical system is your nervous system, and the central heating is your heart and circulation.

If your structure is not sound and the support beams start to tilt, your home will come under increased mechanical pressure. Rather than being able to effortlessly deflect the force of gravity and the stress of the wind, it will start to come under greater strain. Before long the signs of this stress will begin to show. When you look at a building this way, you can appreciate one of the great laws of nature, which is that structure determines function. In other words, the shape of something determines how it works.

When a building has a weak foundation, symptoms of its inability to withstand pressure may begin surfacing as squeaking floor boards, doors that no longer close properly, roof tiles falling, radiators leaking, or cracks appearing in the walls. Your body will respond in a similar way to life's pressures. When faced with an onslaught of symptoms, the obvious thing to do is seek the help of a specialist.

When it comes to your house, you call the carpenter for your floorboards and doors, the plasterer for your walls, and the roofer for your roof. It costs a fair bit of time and money to resolve the issues, but after a few weeks, everything is back to normal—at least as far as you can tell. The symptoms have all been silenced. Winter is just around the corner, however, and just when you don't expect it, a series of storms blow through with gusts of up to eighty mph.

With those storms come unintended consequences such as a year's worth of rain in two weeks.

You batten down the hatches and grit your teeth. You've been through worse, and you know that this period of stress will soon pass. And it does. Spring comes along, and you are excited to open up your house and enjoy it once more. But, to your frustration, the symptoms have all returned. In addition, there's a new large crack down the front wall of your house.

Once again, you call the professionals, but this time, you also call the builder first. After all, the roofer can't repair the wall. He takes a look at it and says, "Look, I can patch that up with some cement and a lick of paint, but the real cause of the problem is in the foundations. You've got subsidence."

When it comes to your body, one of the challenges of modern manual therapies is that there is a professional to call for each area of deterioration. You have a masseuse you see for tight muscles, a physiotherapist for weak muscles, and a chiropractor or osteopath for locked up, misaligned joints and injuries. (These are simplistic explanations. Of course, practitioners within each profession can vary greatly in their approach.) We are served by a broader healthcare system wherein there is a specialist for practically every body part or system. Meanwhile, the holistic way in which all of its parts work together is simply cast aside or outright forgotten.

The problem actually doesn't lie in which practitioner specifically you need to call, but rather how each practitioner thinks about health and the body itself.

Before we go any further, I want to teach you how to do a simple postural assessment on yourself. This will give you some useful insight into how strong your current structural foundation is.

POSTURAL SELF-ASSESSMENT

Stand up. Then, simply breathe in, breathe out, and let your body slump and relax. "Slump" doesn't mean push yourself forwards intentionally, but rather let yourself go where gravity wants you to. You may notice that your shoulders roll inwards, your head and neck come forwards, and there is one or more points in your back where your body appears to "fold" and collapse forwards.

OTHER RESULTS TO LOOK OUT FOR:
- One foot turning out or in more than the other
- One or both feet rolling in
- One hip or shoulder higher than the other
- Pelvis/hips rotated forwards on one side
- Whole body leaning to one side

If you notice any of these results, your structural foundations are not as strong as they should be. You can also do this in front of a long mirror. Stand side-on to it and turn your head slightly so that you can watch your body move. Alternatively, have a partner film you or take a picture so that it is easier to spot the results.

THE SICK CARE SYSTEM

The above analogy of ailing house illustrates the way many people experience their own bodies. We tend to think that everything is okay as long as there are no symptoms on display. True health has a much bigger definition than simply "the absence of symptoms." Being symptom-free is simply one piece of the health puzzle, and to be truly healthy means that you must be in full function, with a strong foundation, able to withstand the stresses and strains of life.

The modern world has become like a pressure cooker, with stress coming at you from all angles. If you are ambitious, you might take on the challenge of running a business or participating in sports—or both. Throw in a family, relationship, and financial pressure on top of that, and your body can become burdened by external pressures that will both create problems and expose a weak foundation. The challenge is knowing how to properly deal with the symptoms as they arrive. This brings us to two distinct and opposing philosophies on health, which are important to know about.

Imagine for a moment that you have a rubber band wound tightly around your finger. As your finger starts to swell, the band becomes tighter, the circulation gets cut off, and your finger begins to hurt. You have two options: take a painkiller, which stops the pain signals from reaching your brain, or find a pair of scissors and cut off the rubber band.

In this example, the painkiller represents a conventional medical approach, also known as allopathy. The cutting off of the rubber band represents a holistic approach. Allopathy seeks to reduce or eliminate the symptoms of the diagnosis (in this case, pain and swelling). Most of conventional mainstream healthcare is allopathic in its approach, which can become very sophisticated. There are several different drugs and that could be used, and there are even advanced testing and surgical techniques that could reduce the swelling in this finger, should it get serious enough.

Holistic care, on the other hand, sees the whole body as one system wherein all parts work together in a self-healing, self-regulating way. It seeks to discover the root cause of health problems and remove the stress on the system, allowing it to get back into homeostasis (a balanced internal state of health). Holistic care, also known as wellness or corrective care, respects that the body is designed to be healthy, and that a state of optimal health is the natural condition for human beings. In the holistic care model, symptoms are recognised as a part of your body's intelligent adaptive response to heal and find balance in the face of lifestyle stresses.

Both of these healthcare models are important and necessary. It is better not to think of either of them as being right or wrong, but rather to think in terms of when it's most beneficial to use each approach.

Imagine that your house is burning down. Who do you call? I hope you said, "The fire brigade." They are the right people to expertly save the life of your house. The firemen have two tools to help you: axes and firehoses, and they will use them to great effect to break down your doors and windows and soak your house with water. This puts out the fire, but in what sort of shape is your house left? It is likely in complete disarray, but it is alive. Thank God.

Now, I ask you, what if your house was in a state of disrepair, the electrical wiring was all wrong, the boiler wasn't working properly, the floorboards were rotting, and the tiles were falling off? The house is miserable, with niggles and dysfunctions everywhere you looked. Who would you call in that case? I hope you said, "Tradesmen and handymen!" These are the people who would come in and redo the wiring, retile the bathroom, replace the floorboards, fix your boiler, and correct the problems with the foundation. They would restore your house to its full glory and make it once again a healthy, functional home.

Once they've done their job, the firemen will often ask, "Don't you know how many houses burn down every year? Don't you know how risky fires are? You should regularly have us visit your house to douse it with water to prevent future fires." This is, of course, metaphorically what the majority of people do. They rely on the firemen (the medical system) with their axes and firehoses (drugs and surgeries) to prevent emergencies.

"What happens to the floorboards, carpets, and walls when they are continuously soaked? Won't they rot? Won't the house be unpleasant to live in?" you'd likely ask.

To which the firemen would respond, "Perhaps, but at least they won't catch fire. You do know how dangerous fires are, don't you?"

And so you wonder about those corrective-wellness experts. Surely, if they were to fix the wiring and restore order, the chances of a fire would be significantly reduced, if not eliminated, right?

"Perhaps," the firemen would respond, "but there is no evidence to prove that is true, so you are better off continuing to beat down the doors and soak your house because we have randomised control trials to prove that this approach works."

Therein lies the problem with the modern health care system: it is largely driven by pharmaceutical companies who control the science and prevailing paradigm. Thankfully, science is quickly evolving, and there is now a plethora of high-quality research that proves, categorically and incontrovertibly, that your lifestyle matters. Your choices with regard to how you move, how you maintain your body structure, how you eat, and how you think have huge impacts on your health as well as the quality of your life and how long you will live. They are the things that really matter.

Here's the bigger challenge: by the time one reaches their teenage years, they've already been exposed to thousands of hours of medical advertising, which teaches them that the way they feel isn't their fault, that their symptoms are a result of bad luck, bad germs, or bad genes. "Just take this pill," they advertise (or, if it's really bad, just have that body part removed altogether), and wait for the symptoms to pass. If you need to keep taking that pill, that's okay. It's better than being bothered by the symptoms, and it's better than having your house burn down. We've been highly trained to think in terms of sickness and symptom reduction rather than health creation.

The prevailing approach says, "If you have a headache, take ibuprofen. If that doesn't work, you can move onto something stronger like codeine, and if that doesn't work, we've got sumatriptan. If that doesn't work, you can bring out the big gun, amitriptyline (an antidepressant), and if that doesn't work...well...just keep taking it anyway, and we can maybe add in some physiotherapy or pain management." I don't mean to sound flippant or to slight the medical approach, I'm simply highlighting the thought process behind the treatment protocol.

The same mentality exists regardless of the condition. Consider chronic high blood pressure, for example. The goal is to lower the blood pressure (reduce the symptom) because it can lead to heart attack and stroke. Treatment is deemed successful when the blood pressure comes down, but what has really happened? One's physiology has been artificially manipulated to change a diagnostic marker, but the patient now needs to continue to take the powerful drug to maintain his symptom-free state. Most often, the underlying cause of the raised blood pressure isn't accurately assessed, addressed, or corrected.

Again, this illustration is somewhat of a simplification because skilled medical doctors will discover or rule out serious causes of high blood pressure and will often recommend lifestyle strategies that can help, but the end result is usually the same: dependence on medication. If you have ever visited your medical doctor with a pain or injury, you likely know firsthand that the first treatment of choice is usually prescribed painkillers. The challenge, however, is that most chronic diseases and pains rarely have a single pathological cause because they are diseases of lifestyle, not medication deficiencies. Also, no imbalance caused by lifestyle errors can ever be corrected with a pharmaceutical drug. It can only be changed, or managed, with the added risk of side effects, which can sometimes be serious.

There are times when the use of drugs may be necessary for the management of symptoms, just ask anyone who has experienced sciatica—pain killers can help to keep them sane whilst further treatment is pursued. However, they shouldn't be relied upon perpetually, or mistaken for true healing, or assumed to be risk free. As I once heard it put so eloquently, "A drug is a poison with a potentially beneficial side effect."

Here's an even simpler way to look at this phenomenon: what would you do if the oil light came on in your car? Would you get a hammer and smash the dashboard? After all, who wants to be distracted by a red light as they drive; smashing it would make it easier not to have to deal with that symptom. Or, would you take your car to a mechanic and have them check out the engine and find out what the issue with the oil is? Of course you'd take it to a mechanic. It's a simple analogy, but it's also a profound one because it helps you think in terms of wellness.

Just like sickness, wellness is simply a lens through which you see the world. It operates off of a different belief system, one that says you are designed to be healthy, that your baseline of operation is peak performance, energy, and health. This is very important because if something goes wrong, your respect for the natural state of health is what will cause you to ask different questions. Rather than try to simply suppress the symptoms, it recognises that the symptoms are a warning sign, and as such, they are also part of the solution. The aches, pains, and annoyances are part of the rebalancing act that was, in fact, allowing you to work at a new— albeit reduced—level of normal.

WHICH WELLNESS PROFESSIONAL DO YOU CALL?

The fundamental difference between allopathy and wellness care is important to understand that it's simply the lens through which you and your healthcare practitioner choose to see health.

Allopathic practitioners (such as general practitioners and Accident & Emergency doctors and surgeons) are the best people to see if your health is experiencing an emergency or life-threatening situation. Thank goodness they are so skilled and proficient in what they do. Yet, when you are looking to restore your health back to its peak state, when you want to get your younger better body back, you need to find a practitioner who operates in the wellness paradigm. They will think beyond symptom suppression to the correction of the cause. That distinction is very important indeed.

Visiting a medical doctor does not guarantee that they will choose to use drugs or surgery; there are many medical doctors who prescribe lifestyle recommendations such as proper diet, nutritional supplements, and exercise rather than drugs. Equally, seeing a chiropractor does not guarantee that they will be thinking holistically. There are many chiropractors, physiotherapists, masseuses, and osteopaths who rely solely on the allopathic paradigm, using natural treatments to put out the little fires of back pain. They are not focused on the whole system or on creating ideal conditions of optimal health and alignment of the whole structure.

The first step to rebuilding your body is learning to think holistically. You must be in relentless pursuit of the fundamental underlying cause of your discomfort so that you can restore long-term balance, not just feel better in the short-term. Restoring structural health requires a lot more than simply rubbing and stretching painful muscles or manipulating stiff joints. While these approaches will often provide pain relief and improved strength and mobility, they won't restore whole body alignment and perfect posture. Restoring your foundation with structural correction demands that you get to the root cause of the imbalance and doing so requires a deeper understanding of how and why body structure goes wrong in the first place.

ALIGNMENT VERSUS POSTURE

Before we can progress further in learning how the body works mechanically, we need to first iron out a common misunderstanding: posture is not the same as alignment. They are related, and are both hugely complicated beasts, but one of them is higher up the priority chain, and that's alignment. Getting clear on the difference between posture and alignment will help you a lot.

THE STRAIGHT TRUTH

Posture is the overall position in which you find yourself in three dimensions when relaxed. It is a complex interplay between your joints, muscles, nervous system, and surrounding environment as they come together make up a particular position. Alignment, on the other hand, which is the more important element here, is the position that something needs to be in in order to work most efficiently.

In terms of health, when anything is operating most efficiently, it is in its most healthy condition. If you have ideal alignment, you will be able to stand effortlessly with what is considered perfect posture. Your body will also function optimally, and you'll be a pain-free, injury-free, high-performance machine. This is why people who are treated with Advanced BioStructural Correction™—even if just for a short timeframe—often report feeling healthier than they have in a long time. There are so many benefits that come from restoring alignment that doing so could be considered to give one an unfair advantage in life, but only because it is lacking in so many. In reality, it is the natural mode of operation.

The struggle between knowing about the importance of good structure and having it show up in your life is real. Many of my patients come to the office already armed with the knowledge that their alignment is far from ideal and has been for a long time. Usually, the conversation goes a bit like this: "My posture is terrible. Always has been. My partner is forever telling me to sit up straight, and I can see in the mirror that my head and shoulders are forwards."

Despite knowing that there is a problem, most people settle into a middle ground where they can see that there is an issue, they would love to fix it, but they've given up hope because they've already tried and failed too many times.

Part of the difficulty is born from the faulty belief that posture is something that you do, rather than something that you have. Trying to hold a "good posture" is, unfortunately, an activity doomed to fail for most people because the moment that one gets distracted, all bets are off. The person soon finds herself back in a slumped position. Since the definition of insanity is doing the same thing over and over while hoping for a different result, it sadly is easy to believe that one is both sane and wise to give up on their quest to be upright.

The prevailing idea is that good posture happens when you stand up straight and pull your shoulders back, but this is not necessarily true, and it's certainly not the whole story. Posture is much more automatic and fundamental to the human frame, and it's a direct result of the alignment of your bones combined with how they interact with one another.

You will come to understand this concept in far greater detail as the book progresses, but most people and practitioners continue to believe the myth that posture is under muscular control, and is therefore corrected by stretching, strengthening, learning new habits and being more conscientious. The truth is, your posture can be changed by those actions, but never truly transformed or corrected. If it were truly corrected, one would naturally stand up straight without any effort. Yet, if you take someone who has worked hard to improve their posture and ask them to stand still, breathe in, breathe out, and let their body relax, you will see their body fold and collapse forwards (either a little bit or a lot) right in front of your eyes. So much for correcting the problem. The root cause of poor alignment was never addressed because it was never understood.

The theory that muscles control your posture can be easily disproved with a simple procedure inside the office of any ABC™ practitioner. The majority of new patients who walk through the door stand with their shoulders rolled forwards (take a look at your family, friends, and colleagues; they will likely all present this way). Standard advice is to hold their shoulders down and back. It's assumed that this solves the problem, but it doesn't. Wait until that person makes a phone call or is distracted in any way; his shoulders will roll forwards again. Yet, when we perform a manual adjustment to their left and right first ribs, restoring the normal alignment of these important bones, the person will immediately take in a deep breath in, their chest will expand more than it did previously, and their shoulders will be effortlessly pinned back into position without any force on the part of the patient. So much for the old idea that muscles are the primary influencer of posture! A poignant quote by Thomas Huxley in 1870 sums it up quite nicely: "The great tragedy of Science—the slaying of a beautiful hypothesis by an ugly fact."

The ugly fact that challenges the current approach of most healthcare professionals is the discovery that the primary driver of posture is bone alignment rather than the action of muscles. And, that when you follow the chain to its logical endpoint, bone alignment is also the primary driver of your body's function. The trouble is, the mechanical function of the human body is not well understood, and this has created a lot of confusion in the world of structural health care. As a result, there is a spinoff of over two hundred techniques in the chiropractic profession alone as well as many different schools of thought on how to correctly restore alignment and balance to the human frame. As you progress through this book you will understand why the discoveries of Dr. Jesse Jutkowitz and the healing science and art of Advanced BioStructural Correction are the solution.

ABC™ is not a theory. It is the practical application of physical laws and engineering principles as they apply to the mechanical life-structure of a human body. This is why it is able to produce predictable and consistent results.

YOUR BODY CAN GET BETTER OVER TIME!

When you first read a statement like that, it's easy to think, "That's just motivational hype; it can't be true." I get it. Conventional wisdom suggests that, as time goes on, our bodies age. It's called degeneration. The trouble is that this belief has become an excuse that allows people to accept their discomfort as "normal" for their age and stage of life. A person with right knee pain suddenly receives the diagnosis of age-related degeneration. Yet, if the degeneration were due simply to age, why doesn't the left knee hurt as well? There is clearly more going on than the onward marching of time.

All too often, pain in the body is chalked up to old age. Patients come in, already labeled with the "age-related degeneration" tag. A person with lower back pain gets an MRI scan and is told that his pain is due to a worn-out or bulging disc, then informed that nothing can be done but accept the reality and take painkillers, maybe try a steroid injection, strengthen their core, and avoid aggravating it. There is almost never even an attempt to try to discover the reason why the joint became a problem in the first place. After all, why bother if it's considered to be caused by old age, bad luck, bad germs, or bad genes?

There is a well-known phenomenon in the world of spinal health wherein a person can present with herniated, degenerated discs on X-rays or MRI scans, yet have no pain. How could that be? The answer is that there is a degenerative process at play within the entire skeleton (not just the spine) that has yet to become enough of a burden to pass the threshold at which symptoms begin or the structure has weakened enough for an injury to occur.

The truth behind most episodes of pain and injury is that there were often many warning signs that were previously ignored. There was a progressive decline in function over time that left someone vulnerable. It's a bit like continuing to put straws on the camel's back; eventually, the final straw causes the poor camel to collapse, but that straw wasn't, in and of itself, the problem. Or tooth decay, where a cavity can often be seen on X-ray as a shadow, months to years before the decay leads to toothache. The cause is clear, though, and unless that hole is filled or the disease process is reversed, the consequences are predictable and inevitable.

There is an underlying and progressive cause at play when body structure fails. It explains and takes into account all manner of body aches, pains, and injuries, from sciatica to headaches to neck pain and beyond. Having posture that is stuck forwards, tight, and twisted is an effect of this cause. You will learn more about this as the book goes on, but one important distinction needs to be made up front is that other problems can exist simultaneously. Health is complex, and there can be many reasons why any particular diagnosis exists. For example, cancers, infections, or fractures can manifest as low back or leg pain. *It is very important to see a qualified professional whenever you have pain so that serious problems can be ruled out.*

Chronic pain is another special case worthy of consideration. Posture plays an important role in cases of chronic and unrelenting body pain. Yet there are other factors that need to be taken into account as well, which I'll discuss further in a bit.

The reason behind the discovery of why bodies degenerate into dysfunction and should come as an exciting concept. Because if we know why it goes wrong and the techniques exist to combat the problem, not only can you correct many of the pains and injuries that have plagued you but you can also regain much of your athletic ability that has potentially been lost over the years.

By working to rebuild your body structure, keeping an active lifestyle, and practicing good nutrition and stress reduction techniques, you can create conditions whereby your body actually improves over time. I can do more now physically and mentally with greater capacity for stress in my mid-thirties than I could in my early twenties. In this day and age, there is no reason why you cannot get better with age by progressively learning the art and science to rebuilding and maintaining a healthy body structure.

YOU CAN'T FIX YOUR OWN POSTURE

It is inarguable that the human body has an incredible capacity for self-healing. It can correct many of its mechanical problems, but not all of them. For example, suppose you fall off your bike and land on your side, causing back pain. Your body will tilt in the opposite direction to compensate for the pain, creating a kink in your spine. Thankfully, you have muscles on the left and right side of your spine as well as on the front of your body that your brain can instruct to contract and pull the spine back into optimal alignment, solving the problem of this misalignment. [See Figure 1A]

However, your spine is the furthest point on the back of your body, which is why you can see and feel the knobbly projections of your vertebrae through your skin. There are no muscles further back from this point, which means that if your spinal vertebrae were to get stuck forwards, there are no muscles available to pull them back into alignment. [See Figure 1B]

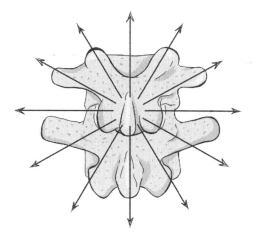

[Figure 1A] Looking at the spine from behind. Muscles can and do attach to the vertebrae in many places that allow the bones to be pulled in many other directions, including forwards but not directly backwards.

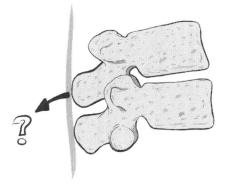

[Figure 1B] Looking at the spine from the side. The most backward part of the spine (known as the spinous process) is right against your skin. There are no muscles attached there that could pull a vertebrae backwards. Even if there were, where would they attach?

This simple fact regarding how the body works is critical to understand. The fact that bones can go out alignment in a direction from which the body has no muscle or combination of muscles to pull in the direction needed to retrieve and replace that bone back into correct alignment explains why posture fails forwards into the slumped position.

You can lean backwards by activating larger muscles of your back (this is actually what happens as part of an intelligent compensation effort by your brain), but you cannot retrieve an individual bone from that forwards, stuck position. A compensated posture will always be less well-off than the original ideally aligned body. Dr. Jutkowitz himself publicly declares that he finds it hard to believe that he was the first person to recognise this fundamental flaw, so to speak, in the human design. Many before him and to this day have simply overlooked the possibility, which is somewhat obvious once you know about it. From this primary injury follows a predictable domino-like chain reaction throughout the skeleton, creating a body-wide, three-dimensional distortion along with all manner of complications. Yet, "complicated" simply means that there are multiple pieces to the puzzle, not that it is indecipherable or impossible to solve. Once you understand what made the primary domino fall, it is possible to run the whole process in reverse and rebuild the human frame with consistency and predictability.

This discovery is a huge advancement in the field of biomechanics and explains why you cannot force good posture upon yourself with conscious muscular effort. Trying to hold yourself upright is doomed to fail in the long-term, no matter how much nagging your mother exposed you to! Pulling your shoulders back, tucking your bum under, lifting your head, and raising your chest may create a better-looking posture, but it is unsustainable. The effort required makes other areas worse, and holding a position that does not match your misaligned bones will exhaust you. As soon as you get distracted, your posture will once again slump back into the configuration that its current state of misalignment allows.

If you do manage to consistently artificially enhance your posture in this way, it will come at a cost by shifting the mechanical problems somewhere else instead. The following experiment will help you to understand:

EXPERIMENT

1. Stand normally without trying to "correct" your posture, and take a deep breath in. Notice the quality of your breath, where the physical restrictions are felt in your chest, how deep it is, how long it is, and how your chest moves.

2. Now, force yourself to stand in the stereotypical perfect posture, as best as you can, by tucking your bum under, lifting your head and chest up to the ceiling, and pulling your shoulders down and back. Take a deep breath in and notice how it feels.

If you correctly followed the instructions, you likely noticed that your breathing was worse off during the second exercise. The exact experience comes down to each person's unique alignment. You probably noticed anything from a slight restriction in depth and quality of breath up to a significant and severe restriction. This is because you mechanically worsened your body by trying to force a better posture, which actually worsened the mechanical function of your joints by adding further complications to the alignment of your spine. The only way you can straighten up without correcting the forwards-stuck bones is by adapting another layer of mechanical stress to your body. This, by the way, is the same reason that posture correction devices are doomed to failure. All of the straps, tapes, elasticated tops, gadgets, and gizmos available to force you upright and pull your shoulders back will make you mechanically worse off, even as they outwardly appear to improve your posture. It usually takes little time before people get tired or something new starts ache, the novelty wears off, and the device goes back in the box.

There is a reason you stand the way you do. Your current posture is the sum total of your body's current best ability and effort to optimise what you've got going on with your alignment and the reality of the mechanical injuries you have accumulated over the years. Generally, the more of these injuries you accumulate, the more distorted from ideal your posture is, the tighter and stiffer your joints are, the more "compensated" your body has become. The human body is incredibly adaptable, but it is equipped with a finite ability to absorb mechanical problems. Eventually, all of the get-out-of-jail-free cards will be used up, and one more injury on top of an already precarious situation can cause people to have chronic pain, injury, and immobility.

THE GRADUAL LOSS OF FUNCTION

It's fascinating to watch children move. We had a two-year-old in the practice a while back watching his mum receive treatment. Out of the corner of my eye, I watched with a smile as he moved around with upright posture, standing tall without any effort. He squatted down with a perfectly straight spine to pick up his milk bottle and remained in that deep squat position ("arse to the grass," as some exercise enthusiasts like to call it). The Asian Squat is a deep squat position commonly used throughout Asian countries in lieu of sitting. This rest position is largely lost in the western world because we spend so much time sitting on chairs and sofas that our bodies get too tight to even get into the position.

He was perfectly relaxed for a couple of minutes as he rested and drank his milk. I smiled because it reminded me of how we should function as human beings. Children are not special cases in terms of how to move, lift, and rest. They simply do what is natural to them because they are not yet burdened by accumulated injuries. It's easy these days to forget what "normal" movement patterns look like and instead simply accept the modern pandemic of dysfunctional bodies as the new normal. We shouldn't, however, confuse common with normal. They are different realities altogether, and a child around the age of two is usually quite a good example of how a human frame should move. All too commonly, unfortunately, that mobility does not last, as one begins to accumulate injuries and dysfunctions throughout modern life.

Later that same morning, another mum brought in her two slightly older children, aged three and five. They immediately headed over to the chairs in the corner and slumped heavily on them, spines and necks curved fully forwards as they stared down at a smartphone and watched YouTube cartoons for the whole session—minds, bodies, and souls transfixed on the screen. This is how postural degeneration begins, partly through learned behaviours, partly through the use of modern furniture (more on how furniture plays a key role in your structural health in Chapter 5) and partly due to unfortunate accidents or injuries that leave a person imbalanced and unable to maintain good alignment. Once that innate sense of upright balance has been lost, a gradual loss of function follows as they spend more and more time fighting the effects of gravity with a forwards-stuck posture.

Whilst you could never say for sure, it is reasonable to suggest that by the time those children are twenty years old, they will have a chronically forwards posture and be suffering the common complaints of neck pain, back pain, and headaches that plague so many adults.

Over the past fifteen years, I have become increasingly convinced that body structure is the biggest kept secret in health care. It is arguably the hardest area of health to address, but also the one from which great benefit can be obtained. As civilisation has become more advanced, we have also become increasing more sedentary and riddled with mechanical problems. This means that there is much to be gained by one's efforts to reverse that trend. Throughout history, from ancient Greeks and Egyptians of 3,000 years ago to modern chiropractors and osteopaths of today, there are records of people recovering from just about everything when the body's alignment is improved.

The health of a body can even be defined by how well that body optimally works on a mechanical basis. This holds true even down to the level of cells, molecules, and atoms for one simple reason: structure governs function.

The question to be asking is not, "Does changing alignment change health?" Rather, it is, "How can we consistently and predictably restore a skeletal frame back to its intended ideal alignment and function?" When you know how to get the foundations of your health corrected and maintained long-term, the optimal level of health and beyond (a state many have come to call one of wellness) is achievable.

Let's take a look at just how far-reaching the effects of your alignment can be.

OLIVER'S UNWINDING STORY

Personal Trainer, Entrepreneur, Author, and Energy Coach, 42

Two years ago, when I first came across Advanced Bio-Structural Correction™, I'd seen some great pictures online of people who had radically improved their posture with ABC™, and I wanted to see if it would work for me. I was struggling with a few things at that point.

Since I'm a personal trainer and health is my passion, I was meant to be an exemplary example of perfect fitness, but I felt that my chest and shoulders were collapsed forwards and I was having to make a real effort to hold myself upright. On top of that, I was getting aches and pains in my back, my neck was restricted moving left and right, and I wasn't feeling like the person I wanted to be.

Once I started my ABC™ treatment, it quickly became apparent that profound changes were starting to happen. My chest came upright, my shoulders to started to come back and drop down, my breathing was improving, and I realised that I was really something of transformation. I noticed that my endurance was improving just going out for runs, and when training clients I wouldn't be audibly breathing at all. My balanced improved with things like squats and lunges and, at the end of the day, instead of being tired and feeling beaten up like I normally would have, I felt loose and had double the energy. And that's really what I've been looking for this whole time.

You've got diet and exercise, which are important, but then you've this third thing: structure. If your structure is in place, your body starts to work the way that it was designed to. And that for me is what's special about ABC™. It's about rebalancing and opening up and just feeling more right with yourself. Your body is back on track and you can depend on it, knowing that you won't wake up in the morning and struggle to get out of bed because yet another new muscle has decided to get stiff and tight. You feel like you did perhaps twenty years ago. I'm still personal training, and I'm in my forties, but I feel, after treatment, no different than I did when I was an athlete (cross country runner) at university in my early twenties.

My flexibility, mobility, balance and appearance have all improved. When I look in the mirror, I'm upright and straight and standing the way that we were meant to stand. I've also just noticed that I've generally been stronger. I've always wanted to work out hard, lift generally heavy weights, and not have to suffer because of it. Now, if I want to, I can deadlift heavy day after day after day and know that I can depend upon my back; it won't give out.

It goes without saying that to anyone sitting on the fence asking, "Should I or shouldn't I do ABC™?" I'd say, "You've just gotta do it! You've got to jump in with both feet!" There's nothing to risk; it's an entirely systematic, progressive, measurable system, and you start to see results straight away. With every visit you get a little bit better and closer to the way your body always should have been operating, which, I suppose, is what we could call our birth right (that is, if we didn't spend ten hours per day hunched over a computer or phone). This is what we should be enjoying, and it's a shame not enough people do.

CHAPTER 2

Alignment Matters

"Get knowledge of the spine, for this is the requisite of many diseases."

—*Hippocrates*

Here's some timeless advice: "Stop slumping; stand up straight with your shoulders back." You've heard it enough times that it might make your eyes roll, but it's not wrong. Since ancient times, the link between good posture, good health, and desirable traits has been recognised and actively pursued. Today's science continues to back up what has been known throughout the ages, clearly showing that posture is a crucial piece of the health and performance puzzle.

In this chapter, we'll take a deep look at the connection between posture, alignment, and health—not only with regard to your physical aches, pains, and injuries but also your systemic health, emotional state, confidence, productivity, quality of mood, and ability to learn and process new information.[1,2] Some studies even show that your posture may influence how long you will remain alive. That's an eye-opening thought! But, at the risk of being an alarmist, alignment really does matter for a whole host of reasons.

Lenon (1994) describes the importance of posture this way:

"Posture affects and moderates every physiologic function, from breathing to hormonal function. Spinal pain, headache, mood, blood pressure, pulse, and lung capacity are among functions most easily influenced by posture."

And,

"Observations of the striking influence of postural mechanics on function and symptomatology have led to our hypothesis that posture affects and moderates every physiologic function from breathing to hormonal function."[3]

Although we understand that good posture is related to good health, many people overlook the ways that poor posture can negatively affect their health. The risk is that pursuing good structural health can be considered (as can exercise) an optional "extra." Yet, we cannot decide to become sedentary and at the same time expect to be healthy. Just as we cannot neglect alignment and then wonder why our overall state of health isn't firing on all cylinders. Adequate movement and proper alignment are critical components of any well-rounded conversation about health.

For ease of discussion throughout the rest of this chapter, I will use the terms *posture* and *alignment* fairly interchangeably, even though they are not technically the same. Much of the research that's been conducted on posture is centred around changing a person's position in space. Amazingly, a simple conscious change of body position can have a pretty profound impact on a person's body and mind. Whereas, in structural correction circles, it is understood that when joint alignment is corrected, posture in the standing and sitting positions are optimised naturally and effortlessly. Good alignment also allows for greatly improved function. Put even more directly, correcting one's alignment unlocks the natural high level of function inherent in all body systems, allowing them to operate at their healthy normal level. Just remember, posture is how something *looks*; alignment is how something *works*.

Unfortunately, as of the time of writing, there are no published studies demonstrating the significant health benefits that are gained through the postural transformation following treatment with ABC™. This methodology is an emerging discipline, and whilst several exciting research studies have begun throughout the world, we are still awaiting their publication. This is why I have cited existing studies on posture. Even though they are incomplete, they still give incredible insight into the power that alignment holds over your health.

PHYSICAL ROBUSTNESS AND PERFORMANCE

Take a look at any high-performing athlete, and you will quite clearly notice that they have an upright and symmetrical body. You're not going to see a champion sprinter standing on the start line with his neck jutted forwards like a chicken. The fact is, you are highly unlikely to be able to perform at a high level physically if your body's mechanics are not in good working order. On the other hand, you rarely see someone suffering from chronic poor health or injuries whose posture is not also suffering from postural degeneration and, most commonly, the classic "stuck forwards" position.

The way in which your body is arranged in space forms the foundation that determines how well you will move and how well you can to adapt to the stresses of life. Imagine trying to lift a 50 kg box with a curved back, or playing tennis with your chin on chest, or even just sitting in an awkward posture for ten minutes. Some part of your body is very likely to start hurting. It is, therefore, clear that we function better—and *feel* better—when our joints are aligned to meet the needs of the task at hand.

The simple reason alignment matters so much is that, during every moment of your life, you are exposed to a constant and unrelenting force that is potentially devastating to your body. Ironically, life on Earth could not exist without this force because it acts as the glue that holds everything together. I am, of course, talking about gravity.

The force of the Earth's gravitational field is continuously pulling you down towards the Earth's surface at a force of approximately 608 newtons (assuming you weigh 62 kg). This means that whenever you are upright, either standing or moving about, your joints are being placed under gravitational load. Your body works mechanically as a complex series of levers, and we know that the longer the lever is, the greater the force we can generate with it. If you are standing up correctly and in ideal alignment, there should be nothing but direct compression placed evenly throughout all the weight-bearing bones of your body, which you are more than capable of dealing with. If you have a forward-stooped posture, however, you have a lever in your spine upon which gravity pulls. The more forwards your head is, the longer the lever is, and the greater the force that's placed on your neck, back, and rest of your body.

You can easily imagine the extra force this places on your body structure with a simple mind experiment. Imagine that your head were a bowling ball (a human head and a bowling ball weigh about the same amount, around 5kg). If you were to hold the bowling ball in the palm of your hand above your shoulder, you could probably hold it there for quite some time. Now imagine how much harder it would be to hold that bowling ball out *in front* of your shoulder, even if it were just six inches forwards of the midline. There is a significant difference, because of the addition of a lever.

Research shows that for every inch your head gets stuck forwards, it gains 4.5kg in weight, as far as the muscles of your neck and back are concerned. They have to work harder to stop your head from collapsing to your chest. This extra effort is occurring throughout your body, not just on your neck muscles. So, the important point to grasp here is that if your posture is off, your entire structure has to work harder (and less efficiently) in order to keep you balanced and injury-free.

In the stuck-forwards posture, some muscles will become tight whereas others may become weak and inhibited, a phenomenon easy to demonstrate through muscle testing in a clinical setting or by observing the way that someone gets up from a chair or by their form in the gym. Over time, these abnormal adaptations harm a body's ability to resist the forces placed upon it, inflicting extra wear and tear on joints, ligaments, and muscles, increasing the likelihood of classic aches, pains, and injuries associated with life and sports. Name any issue involving physical pain; it can probably be traced to the impact of poor posture or too much time in improper positions. Researchers have linked poor posture to scoliosis, tension headaches, back pain, neck pain, and so on. Although it's not necessarily the exclusive cause of any of them, it is a direct and significant contributing factor in many cases, including the difficult beast that is chronic pain.

THE CHRONIC PAIN CONUNDRUM

Chronic pain is defined as pain that persists or progresses over a long period of time, usually several months or years. Examples are sciatica, arthritis, and migraine headaches. Whilst some studies show that poor posture can lead to chronic pain and affect sensitivity of pain,[4] there are other studies that show a poor correlation between the two. The reason for this is twofold. First, good posture is not necessarily synonymous with good mechanics. A person can appear to be relatively upright but still have a lot of joint, muscle, and nerve dysfunction going on beneath the surface. We see this in practice quite often with the bolt upright military spine. Whilst this can appear at first glance to be a "good" posture, the mechanical reality underneath the surface is one of poor alignment, and it's highly compromised. There is much disagreement as to the best way to correct joint alignment, but as I will show you in the next chapter, the lack of a consensus is based on the fact that the underlying reason posture fails has only recently been discovered; it's not yet widely known. Second, pain can be a tricky beast and have tentacles that spread into many aspects of a person's health. The biopsychosocial model of pain[5] is one of the more comprehensive theories that attempts to explain the true complexity of pain. Essentially, it shows that emotional stress, traumas, injuries, illnesses, nerve damage, and other physical problems in the body can cause pain. Psychological factors such as anxiety, depression, mood, and fear also play a role, as do social factors such as relationships, work, occupation, and isolation.

Most doctors and all body structure-based practitioners are in agreement that good posture is the most desirable and healthy structural condition for a human being. I don't hear anyone arguing the case that we should pursue poor posture. I do, however, hear some throwing the baby out with the bath water on the back of research that suggests that posture doesn't correlate one hundred percent with pain. This is no reason to cast aside the pursuit of a more ideal human frame, both for the lack of completeness those sorts of conclusions are based upon (the lack of correct joint alignment for one) and the fact that the mechanical functioning of the body is one of many important contributing factors that still needs to be addressed in cases of complex and chronic pain.

WHAT IS GOOD POSTURE, ANYWAY?

If you take a look at the people around you at work or on the streets, you will likely notice that very few people have what is considered to be "good posture." The general scientific consensus is that the more sedentary we have become, the worse the effect has been on our physical bodies. The effects of computer and commuter generations have turned the once upright homosapien into a new species, the "round-shouldered homo-sedentarien."

It's one thing to look at the problem, but what is the solution? What should an ideal posture look like? This is a surprisingly complicated question to answer because posture varies depending upon what you are doing. Let's start by remembering what good posture is *not*. It's not about simply engaging your muscles and rearranging your joints so that you stand up tall with your shoulders back. Amazingly, this is what most people—including researchers on the subject—think defines good posture. In their defense, they are partly correct, but there is so much more going on beneath the surface in terms of the ways in which all of a person's bones interact.

Trying to create good posture in this way is a bit like buying a fake Rolex watch. Whilst it may look like the real thing and fool onlookers at first glance, when a trained eye takes a closer look, all sorts of imperfections become clear. A real Rolex, on the other hand, not only looks flawless on the outside, it is also significantly more valuable for the simple reason that the intricate internal mechanical cogs are perfectly engineered, perfectly aligned, and flawless in their mechanism, running smoothly without stress or strain. An original Rolex maintains its value; some even go up in value over time. This is the way the human frame is designed to work to a certain degree. Oftentimes, when I look at the classic follow-up "transformation" pictures that you find online of people who have been through a program of postural exercises involving stretching and strengthening rehabilitation work, the person looks strained (with their tummy tucked in, shoulders pulled back, and head held up into extension, for example). It is clear that it takes effort to maintain their new 'improved' posture, which is not sustainable, and as you will learn in the next chapter, this effort actually creates a new set of problems for the body to deal with mechanically. Aging will eventually get the better of each of us, but if we look after our alignment, we can continue to enhance our physicality for multiple decades, maintaining great function and improving skills into our seventies, eighties, and perhaps beyond. In that way, we can be like a real, rare-edition Rolex watch.

Good posture is not a static concept. For example, the ideal posture for someone doing a standing bicep curl is different from the ideal posture for someone doing a handstand or pushing something heavy overhead. It's different yet again for someone doing a deadlift or squat. Each of these movements and positions requires a different body posture. The bones need to move and align correctly to allow for natural strength of form in whatever activity one is engaged in. If you are out of alignment thanks to previous injuries or lifestyle errors, you may be unable to get yourself in the correct posture to be able to correctly perform a specific movement. This is when injury can occur.

The scientific field that studies how joints and muscles interact in order to produce movement in the human body is called biomechanics. This is a term that you will often hear thrown around quite loosely. It's not uncommon, for example, to hear someone utter the phrase, "You need to improve your biomechanics." This is technically inaccurate, and what the person really means to say is that you need to improve your alignment so that your body can work in a more mechanically efficient and correct way. We have already learned that improving muscles (by stretching, strengthening, activating, pushing needles into, or electrocuting them) will not achieve this because *bones can go out of place in directions that the body has no muscles or combination of muscles to pull them in the direction needed to return to their optimal position.* This is such a crucial point that it bears repeating.

You can temporarily improve some of your body mechanics by forcing some motion or position of your body, as a tennis player works to plant his foot in a certain way to have a better swing, but it will always be at the expense of some other area or areas of his body mechanics, which will worsen. This is the same reason that forcing yourself to hold a better posture is tiring and reduces the effectiveness of your breathing. You traded one mechanical problem for another.

The main goal of structural correction is to restore proper alignment and mechanical function to the body, not teach a person to hold a "good posture." Understood in this way, posture becomes a way of keeping score, so to speak, because the natural consequence of correcting alignment is that, in a relaxed standing position, a person will *effortlessly* assume an ideal posture, without needing any muscular effort to do so. For the same reason, athletes all over the world are discovering that ABC™ is making it much easier for them to get their bodies in the correct positions for their sport and are performing much better and more easily as a result.

In Figure 2 you can see what an ideal posture should look like. Each of the numbered points need to line up absolutely correctly for your joints to work in optimal mechanical flow with minimal degeneration. They are not approximations; remember that alignment refers to the position a joint needs to be in to function properly.

It is fascinating to recognise that ailments many consider to be major, incurable diseases are commonly the effect of poor alignment—for example, points 1, 2, and 4 not lining up vertically. If given the choice, would you rather have lower back surgery or go through a corrective care process that gets these points lined up correctly again? Chronic headaches? I'd check whether points 1 and 2 were lining up correctly. Chronic shoulder impingement or rotator cuff syndrome? Look at points 2, 3, 9, and 12. Carpal tunnel syndrome or tennis elbow? Look at points 9, 10, and 11. Wear and tear on the knee? Patellar tracking disorder? Look at points 4, 5, and 6. This approach is certainly a lot more convenient than a knee replacement, wouldn't you say? The physics of the body are really fascinating, but we must remember that you cannot look at one part in isolation. Points 1 to 18, along with many others, all work together as one complete synchronised system. Understanding of that one key point is why ABC™ is able to be so consistently effective.

In this ideal relaxed and optimally aligned state, when you look at the posture from the front or the back, all twenty-four vertebrae should appear stacked in a straight line. From the side, one should have three curves: one in the neck, one at the mid-back, and one at the small of the back. You aren't born with all three curves. Babies usually have just one C-shaped curve. The others develop around twelve to eighteen months as the muscles strengthen while the baby learns to stand and walk and spends more time upright.

If you are ideally aligned, when you are standing up you should be able to draw a straight plumb line from your ear hole through the middle of your shoulder, middle of your hip, middle of your knee, and ankle joint.

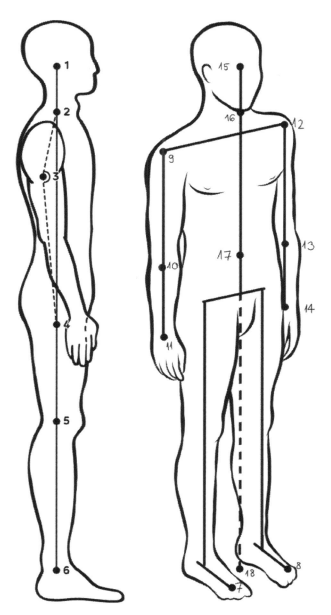

[Figure 2] Ideal posture in a perfectly aligned and relaxed body.

This keeps your centre of gravity directly over your base of support, which is centred between your feet, under your pelvis. Each of your feet has three arches that provide you with structural support, but your feet, legs, and pelvis also work together to form one large arch. Along with your spinal curves, your feet spread the weight evenly and effectively through a comprehensive system of natural levers that keep you upright with minimal muscular effort.

If you are not correctly aligned, your bone lever system will fail to work efficiently and muscles will have to tighten to support you against the onslaught of gravity. This muscular effort can make it appear as if your posture is okay, when in fact, it is off.

This is why it is important to ensure that a person is completely relaxed when assessing their posture. Otherwise, the true posture of the person is not revealed. In my practice, we use the instruction, "Breathe in; breathe out; let your body slump and relax." It is fascinating to witness that, even after the first session of structural correction, a person will find it almost impossible to slump (unless they physically push themselves forwards) for the simple reason that they have regained the mechanical leverage that comes from correct alignment. When an ABC™ practitioner adjusts you, your breathing comes online, the room brightens, your shoulders are naturally down and back, and you feel perfectly balanced and symmetrical. It feels as though you are lighter and you float out of the room with a lovely sense that your body is effortlessly working for you rather than against you.

One of the interesting relationships that I have noticed amongst patients who have been through our structural correction programs is that they regularly report an improvement in energy as they come out of the forwards-stuck position into a better posture. This makes perfect sense when you consider that if you are out of alignment, your body has to constantly expend extra energy to combat the effects of gravity.

Roger Sperry, Ph.D. (Nobel Prize winner in Physiology of Medicine 1981) spent a lifetime studying functional neurology and describes the drain of poor posture this way:

"Better than ninety percent of the energy output of the brain is used in relating the physical body in the gravitational field. The more mechanically distorted a person is, the less energy is available for healing metabolism and thought."

When you consider that many people work desk jobs where their heads are pushed forwards and their spines are slumped for many hours each day, you can appreciate just how much energy is wasted in order to simply hold oneself upright, not to mention the tightness and achiness that comes alongside that expended energy[6]. On their website, the NHS even lists poor posture as one of the main energy stealers and causes of fatigue,[7] and surgical procedures have been improved in the past so that surgeons can maintain better ergonomics and reduce the effects of fatigue[8].

POSTURE IS A PROCESS

In this chapter I have outlined the ideal scenario for posture, but it is important to understand that rebuilding your body and restoring ideal posture is a process that occurs over time. You won't get to the ideal scenario pictured in Figure 2 (below) overnight. We call the posture transformation process "unwinding" (you will learn all about unwinding in Chapter 4). As a body unwinds, there are many subtle clues and signs of progress that experienced ABC™ practitioners look out for. Straightening up is only one of them. Posture is a much bigger conversation than one in which only how upright someone is matters. Whilst bodies do straighten up significantly, quickly, and completely, given enough good treatment with ABC™, for many people their mechanical problems are too complex to allow that to happen immediately. This is why, when you see a picture on social media of someone with their back and head arched into extension, their tummy sucked in all the way, and their shoulders forced down and back, you can confidently say, "Uh oh, that person is actually worse off than they were before." Much of what is available to help posture is superficial, temporary, and incomplete. Yet, if you buy into the notion that looking straighter is the only goal, you will miss the bigger picture and result of a body that works well mechanically.

Here are some of the key observation points that we use to assess how good a patient's posture really is.

- *Smoothness of the three spinal curves:* A poorly aligned body will have flat spots as well as twists and sharper, angular points of transition between the backwards and forwards curves of the spine. These curves become smoother and broader after a good session and continue to improve over time until eventually the normal curves and symmetry are restored.
- *Points of postural collapse/folding:* Forwards-stuck spinal bones cause varying degrees of "folding" in the spine as a person breathes out. This phenomenon disappears when ABC™ is applied correctly, and the patient will be stable and relaxed on breathing out.
- *Balancing out:* A misaligned body is stuck in a twisting/tilting pattern head to toe. You will see ears, shoulders, and hips all become more balanced when adjusted with ABC™.
- *Better breathing:* The depth, symmetry, and smoothness of rib and chest movement on breathing.
- *Skin colour and tone:* Good alignment affords optimal blood flow, and a person's skin tone will very often go from pale to flushed/vibrant.
- *Head position:* When the lower neck bone (C7) is correctly aligned, the natural C-shape curve of the neck is returned, and this shift is readily observable. Interestingly, the plane of the

face should be perpendicular to the ground. If you see the face angled down, that's not a good thing because it means that something, probably C7, is stuck forwards. Equally, if you see the face angled upwards, it means that they are being held in extension with compensation effort. This is also not good and doesn't happen in a body that is being optimally corrected with ABC™.

- *Chest shape:* There should be no inwards curving or scalloping of the upper chest. Even after one session of ABC™, you will notice that the chest looks fuller and opens up. The scalloping improves or goes away. Often, the chest will also go from stuck and rigid to flexible and mobile as it improves.

- *Abdominal shape:* When the lower back bones, particularly L5, are stuck forwards, the lower abdomen can poke further forwards, particularly the section beneath the belly button. When the lower back is correctly aligned, this little pooch disappears, and a person can visibly look "thinner." With ideal alignment, the belly button is the most forwards point on the abdomen, not the area below it.

- *Stillness:* Any jerking or wobbling on breathing (points of major mechanical tension and misalignment often appear very rigid and can cause a noticeable jerky motion or wobble as a person breathes). A very imbalanced structure can also lead to an ongoing and body-wide wobble, where a person is constantly shifting their body position in an attempt to get stable. These "wobbly" bodies often have a lot of mechanical issues and improve tremendously with ABC™ over time.

- *Shoulder position:* Ideally, shoulders should be naturally and effortlessly down and back. When the first rib is misaligned, the shoulder will roll forwards upon breathing out, which is readily observable.

- *Arm and hand positions:* You should see only the thumb and first finger when standing directly in front of a person. If you can see the back of the hand it means that there is misalignment and compensation twisting going on. Equally, the gaps between the elbows and the abdomen should be equal and symmetrical.

- *Leg and feet positions:* Often, one foot is turned out further than the other, one or both foot arches appear flattened and/or one or both knees can be rolled in or hyper-extended. The feet can be planted too far apart to maintain stability with a broader base. Each of these factors improves and balances out with unwinding.

- *Face symmetry:* Interestingly, even the face can give clues as to what is happening with a person's alignment and mechanical function. Again, symmetry is the key factor that we are looking for. One eye that appears squinted, a jaw that is off to either side, uneven wrinkles, and a sort of strained tension throughout the facial muscles can all be important clues of misalignment, and believe it or not, these also improve as unwinding progresses.

BEING STUCK FORWARDS COULD BE AN OVERALL HEALTH PROBLEM, NOT JUST A BACK PROBLEM

As posture degenerates forwards, there is a gradual twisting and tightening of the skeleton that occurs, leading to the potential for pain or injury from your head to your feet. Organs do not escape the physical strain either. Your chest and abdomen are essentially cavities that are filled with squidgy bits such as a heart, lungs, and intestines, which may get compressed, stretched, or otherwise distorted when posture collapses forwards.

Lenon *et al* 2004 state that:

"The most significant influences of posture are upon respiration, oxygenation, and sympathetic function. Ultimately, it appears that

homeostasis (body in balance) and autonomic regulation (automatic functions) are intimately connected with posture."[3]

Lung function in particular, which is a directly influenced by chest function, is easily affected by changes in posture.[9] You can prove this to yourself by sitting upright and taking a deep breath in, then comparing that to the depth and quality of breath you can draw in when in a fully slumped position. It's very clear that we breathe better when we aren't slumped forwards. Being stuck forwards puts a physical restriction on your spine, ribs, and muscles of respiration—particularly your diaphragm, which is a hugely important muscle that performs many crucial tasks.

Your diaphragm is the primary muscle of respiration, but it is also intricately linked to other body functions such as your autonomic nervous system, within which conscious control of breathing can help regulate your stress response. It has a role in controlling posture and stabilising your trunk during exercise, and also in helping the heart function given its influence on chest pressure and the way in which blood flows in and out of your heart. This important muscle is also closely linked to lymphatic drainage as well as helping to form an anatomical barrier against acid reflux from your stomach.[10] You definitely want to keep your diaphragm in good working order.

If you understand the principle of hydraulics, you can quickly grasp how breathing should ideally occur. Your diaphragm is the primary breathing muscle. It's a thin, dome-shaped muscle that separates your chest cavity from your abdominal cavity. When the diaphragm contracts, the diaphragm's dome shape flattens out and pushes downwards onto your abdominal organs, like a piston in a cylinder. This creates a reduction in chest pressure, which allows air to be drawn into the lungs, causing them to expand.

Your diaphragm is attached to the underside of your ribs as well as your spine and sternum. When it contracts, there is an expansion of your rib cage and belly in all directions. In other words, if your diaphragm is working correctly, you will expand like a barrel. This is how we *should* breathe, yet because of the proliferation of forwards stuck bodies and sedentary lifestyles, many people's joint mechanics don't allow for optimal diaphragm function. A stiff and forwards spine compresses the diaphragm and adds resistance to its movement. Whilst it still contracts, its function is reduced, and it can become weak, deconditioned, and lazy over time. This causes many people to use what are known as accessory muscles of respiration. Muscles of the neck, back, and shoulders can help with breathing, particularly during intense exercise, but they shouldn't take over the job long-term. Over time, chronic neck and upper chest breathing can exhaust and potentially damage these accessory breathing muscles, leading to whole host of potential problems.

One such problem is the development of painful nodules known as trigger points. You have probably felt these as painful bumps in your neck and shoulder muscles. They usually sit there dormant, but if you stress them too much, they can become active and send pain throughout your back, head, shoulder, and arms. The pain can be significant, and the traditional treatment—which involves putting heavy pressure on the muscle knot—is equally unpleasant.

The more you stress your neck and shoulder muscles through poor breathing, the greater the likelihood you will develop both acute and chronic injuries of the neck and shoulders. This includes ailments such as thoracic outlet syndrome, frozen shoulder, rotator cuff impingements, and chronic neck pain.[11] There is also the obvious issue of fatigue associated with poor breathing due to the potential for reduced oxygen uptake to the brain and other organs. Shallow breathing may also activate the sympathetic nervous system, leading to a chronic activation of that system's fight or flight response. Chronic stress has, of course, been linked to nearly all chronic diseases and is certainly one of the key aspects of health to keep under control. Feelings of stress and anxiety are intimately related to how well you breathe. Just ask anyone who regularly meditates how effective diaphragmatic breathing is at calming down both their body and mind. Equally, you will not see someone who is panicked or anxious taking deep, slow, diaphragmatic breaths. Instead, they will be taking short, sharp, and fast breaths through the upper chest. Restoring optimal breathing may be one of the best ways to help combat the effects of the fast-paced, stressful modern world. Poor breathing also impacts one's desire to actually get up and do the things that matter, like exercise. The burn of working out is unpleasant enough without the added drag of inefficient breathing and the tight neck, back, and shoulders that follow.

The proverbial cat seems to be out of the bag when it comes to the importance of good breathing. There are many different breathing exercises that can help, such as lying on your back with a book on your chest and trying to elevate it towards the ceiling as you breathe. Restricted breathing through tubes, breath holding exercises, box breathing, and many other tips and tricks can be explored. Disciplines like yoga teach people to become better breathers by focusing on diaphragmatic breathing. With practice, patience, and time, it's possible to improve the function of your own diaphragm and the quality of your breathing. The main downside to these approaches, which I've observed in countless patients over the years, is the tendency to become fixated on one's breath. This leads them invariably to 'over breathe' which can set up all sorts of physiological imbalances in the body. One of the best resources I can recommend on learning to breathe correctly is *The Oxygen Advantage* by Patrick McKeown. If you recognise that your breathing needs to be improved, or if you suffer from a respiratory condition or want to improve sports performance, fine-tuning this essential life function could really help.

The important distinction to make, however, is that quality breathing shouldn't necessarily have to be consciously controlled; it is under the influence of the autonomic nervous system, which means that it should merrily get on with its job without you ever having to think about it. This is where structural correction can once again save the day. It has a significant impact upon chest function, which directly affects the way that you breathe. When the spine and ribs are correctly positioned, the diaphragm automatically comes back online. Once the mechanical tension has been removed, the breath is deep and easy. Interestingly, the result can be seen throughout almost the entire body. When a person is mechanically sound and breathing well, you can see the chest, abdomen, and even lower back expand equally and effortlessly as they breathe. The main point is that this happens automatically without the need to re-educate one's breathing technique. An important concept to remember is that *your body rarely needs any help to function well; it just needs no interference.*

With so many functions of your health tied to your breathing, it should come as little surprise that lung function has been closely linked to longevity. Several studies have shown that lung function is arguably the best predictor of mortality in the general population, meaning that if your lung function declines, your risk of dying increases. The authors of one twenty-nine-year-long follow-up study concluded that "it is surprising that this simple measurement (the amount of air you can forcibly exhale in one second) has not gained more acceptance as a general health assessment tool, including testing for life insurance."[12] For this reason, I track the lung function of my patients with a digital spirometer and almost universally see improved readings, even after just one ABC™ adjusting session.

There are other studies that have made compelling mortality links along similar lines. Kado et al[13], for example, demonstrated that people with a hyperkyphotic (stuck forwards) posture had a forty-four percent increased death rate. This means that an increasing kyphotic posture is tied to an increasing all-cause mortality, which essentially determines one's chances of dying from any health condition. In particular, it is associated with a 2.4 times greater chance of dying from atherosclerosis, a serious disease where arteries gradually clog up and harden. Another finding of this study was that hyperkyphosis was *not* found to be correlated with osteoporosis, which is the classic condition wherein a gradual softening of the bones leads to compression fractures and a serious rounding of the mid back, particularly in the elderly. This is an important point because it confirms that the health consequences of a forwards stooping body are due to a mechanical change, which can be improved with possible life-extending effects. On the other hand, the forwards stooping that comes with osteoporotic vertebral fractures is a difficult problem to treat, and usually cannot be stopped without risky surgery. These osteoporotic patients can still be safely treated with ABC™ to help with pain and mobility, but they will always be at a mechanical disadvantage due to the wedged shape of any fractured vertebrae.

This isn't just a one-off finding. Several other large studies have also demonstrated that a forwards-stuck posture is linked to worsened health, including impaired lung function, poor physical function, reduced quality of life, greater risk of falls and fractures, and higher mortality rates.[14, 15, 16] Along similar lines, the British Regional Heart Study followed a large group of men over a twenty-year time span and found that those who lost 3cm in height were sixty-four percent more likely to die from a heart attack. They also found that those men who lost an average of 1.67 cm were associated with a forty-two percent increased risk of heart attacks.[17] The authors gave a few suggestions as to why this happens, from muscle loss to osteoporosis and reduced nutritional status, all of which could be involved. Yet, I would argue that it is easy to overlook the importance of having good posture throughout life on one's long-term health. It is just one factor, but it's a crucial one.

There is a mechanical explanation for the impact of poor posture on cardiovascular health. Your heart, as amazing as it is, is essentially a mechanical muscular pump. Once it has contracted and squeezed out all the blood, it elastically recoils and expands into the chest cavity. The more it expands, the more blood can be taken onboard and pumped out in the next contraction. If poor posture causes the chest cavity to become compressed, rigid, and narrowed, the heart is less able to fully expand due to the reduced space and takes on less blood as a result. In order to pump the required volume of blood around the body, the heart then has to work harder with a reduced stroke volume and pumping capacity, which raises blood pressure and pulse rate.

There are many ways that a person's posture can distort. Sometimes they fall forwards, sometimes they straighten out in mid back, but mechanically they are all part of the same mechanism (covered in detail in next chapter). A back that straightens out is sometimes referred to as a military spine or as straight back syndrome. The mechanical impact of this sort of posture on your heart and lungs is easier to comprehend because the chest cavity becomes thinner, and there is visibly less room for the heart and lungs to expand. Many studies from the 1960s to 1980s looked at this link and related it to health problems such as heart murmurs and respiratory distress or failure. [18, 19]

There are potential neurological links between posture and blood pressure as well. A 2007 study out of Leeds University revealed that hours spent hunched over a computer with poor posture may raise one's blood pressure. Scientists found a direct neural connection between the neck muscles and a part of the brainstem called the nucleus tractus solitarius (NTS), which is known to help regulate heart rate and blood pressure.[20]   Granted, they were studying mice, but the connection nevertheless provides an interesting new understanding of how a chronic forwards-stuck posture (which places a lot more mechanical strain on the neck muscles) could, in theory, play an important role in cardiovascular health. This potential relationship is further supported by studies showing a reduction in blood pressure following manipulation of neck vertebrae (McKnight and DeBoer, 1988, Knutson 2001).

With the limited research available, we have to be careful with the way that conclusions are drawn between posture and systemic health. Posture correction cannot, at this stage, be considered as a treatment for any chronic health condition since such conditions are complex, multi-system problems with many possible confounding variables. The aim to improve posture should not be considered a treatment for any particular condition since diet, stress, smoking, obesity, poor fitness, toxicity, hormones, structure, and (to a certain degree) genetics can all play important contributing roles. Rather, seeking an improved posture should be an attempt to return the body back into a physical state of ease. Once back in mechanical balance, the body has a better chance of functioning optimally and re-finding health.

AS IN SPINE SO IN MIND; YOUR POSTURE AND YOUR THOUGHTS

We've talked about peak athletic performers having a good posture. Well, if you see an Olympic sprinter win the gold medal, you will also see her strut around with great poise—head held high, shoulders back, chest inflated, demonstrating an air of unshakeable confidence. We know that confident people hold themselves well, and interestingly, in sports and in life, if a good posture helps you to succeed, you have a positive feedback cycle set up that helps you go from one success to the next.

On the other side of the spectrum, people who are depressed and lacking confidence tend to demonstrate slumped-forwards postures. Your emotional patterns and attitudes towards life appear to be hardwired into the neurology of your movement patterns. Here's an experiment to help you recognise how your emotional state is connected to your posture:

EXPERIMENT

Sit in a chair and let your chin come to your chest, your shoulders roll inwards, and your back slump. Notice how you feel. This is a contracted physical state, and you will probably feel downcast, saddened, defeated, or even depressed. Next, sit up really tall, lift your head high, and raise your arms up, turning your palms towards the sky. In this expanded state, you will probably want to take a deep breath in and will find it hard to keep the smile from your face. This is the confident, happy feeling that comes with an optimal posture.

Humans as well as animals tend to express power and confidence through open, expansive postures. Think of a gorilla standing tall and beating his chest or a lion roaring with his chest puffed out. Humans do it too. Displays of confidence and dominance can be achieved non-verbally by raising our chest and pulling our shoulders back, placing our hands on our hips (think Superman). Not that people really think about it, it's just part of what we do. Yet, you could use it to your advantage if you wanted to because research shows that if you deliberately assume one of these so-called power postures for just a few seconds, you will physiologically experience elevations in testosterone, reductions in cortisol, and an increased feeling of power and tolerance for risk. [21, 22] Another study showed that posing in a positive, upright posture led individuals to rate themselves higher in leadership ability than did posing in a negative, slouched posture. [23] This is potentially useful information if you are ambitious and looking to make strides forward in life. Equally, if you lack confidence, knowing that a simple shift in your posture could help you feel more like a confident, powerful leader (and be perceived that way by others) could be of great help. From a health perspective, this is also useful to know because upright, dominant, power postures have been linked to an increased tolerance to pain. [24]

It appears that the full complexity of the way we're able to show up day to day may very well go beyond just our thoughts and feelings, and merge into the way that we move and hold ourselves. We innately understand this, since we're able to read someone's emotional state simply by analysing their body posture and facial expressions. It's clear, for example, what someone is thinking if they roll their eyes at your humble, helpful suggestion. Or, if you sit with your arms and legs crossed, it's considered a defensive posture whereby you're giving off clues that you feel uncomfortable or threatened by your present situation.

If your body language speaks, it stands to reason that your posture does as well, even when facial expressions and situational clues are taken out of the equation. Researcher Mark Coulson showed that there is almost universal recognition of the posture of sadness, where the head is bent forwards by about fifty degrees and the back is curved into a C-shape. Similarly, surprise, happiness, and anger highly correlated with certain postures, so we have a certain ability to correctly determine emotional states from the human frame alone.[25] Posture, therefore, has become part of the way we assess and understand the expression of emotions through body language. It is interesting to think that even though we express ourselves through words, a link between one's physical posture and mental emotional state can be seen. The term "attitude" for example, originally referred to a person's physical posture, but it now has multiple meanings with regard to one's opinion *and* behaviour. Today, people often use the term *position* or *posture* to refer to their opinion on an issue. Given this two-way relationship, an interesting question to ask is: if emotions can distort posture, can posture distort emotions?

The conclusion is not, however, as simple as "good posture equals positive emotions, and bad postures equals negative emotions." Posture may simply be more dynamically intertwined into the way that we process our experience of life. A 2009 study from The Ohio State University looked at this deeper relationship in more detail. Students were asked to think about and write down their best or worst qualities while they were either sat up with their back erect and their chest pushed out (confident posture) or slouched forwards with their back curved (doubtful posture). The end result was that when students wrote positive thoughts about themselves, they rated themselves more highly when sat upright than when slumped because the the upright posture led to confidence in their positive thoughts. Interestingly, however, when the students wrote negative thoughts about themselves, they rated themselves more negatively when they were in an upright rather than a slouched posture, again because the upright posture led to more confidence in their thoughts. This trend demonstrates that in a confident, upright position, we give more power to our thoughts when forming self-attitudes, whereas in a doubtful, slumped posture, we tend to allow our thoughts to judge ourselves to a lesser degree.

In a separate experiment, researchers asked the students a series of questions about how they felt during the course of the study. "These participants didn't report feeling more confident in the upright position than they did in the slumped position even though those in the upright position did report more confidence in the thoughts they generated."[26] The takeaway is that in the upright position you are more confident in your thoughts, no matter what they are, so your thoughts are likely influenced by your posture whether you realise it or not.

Another study looked into the idea that postures are not merely passive indicators of the way you are feeling, but they can also affect both a person's mental state and behaviour. The researchers took a group of students and had them perform an aptitude test. They were then asked to perform a second short experiment wherein they were delivered a note that either said they were very successful (top twenty percent) or had been very unsuccessful (bottom twenty percent) compared to their peers. Participants were then randomly assigned to a slumped or upright position for eight minutes, after which they were taken to another room to complete an unsolvable geometric puzzle. The results of the experiment showed that when a slumped posture was "inappropriate" to the current situation (i.e. they had just succeeded), the slumping seemed to undermine subsequent motivation as well as feelings of control. But when "appropriate" (i.e. they experienced failure), slumping minimised feelings of helplessness and depression as well as motivation deficits. This means that a slumped posture may help people to better process negative events, but it will leave them feeling less in control and able to take advantage of positive events. By the same token, an upright posture helps people process positive situations well, but it could leave them more depressed in the face of negative outcomes. These results strongly suggest that we use posture to help guide and moderate information processing and our responses to good and bad events of everyday life.[27]

Research findings such as these certainly raise an important point for consideration in an age when the average person's posture is getting worse rather than better. While posture can be influenced moment-to-moment with conscious effort, if there are existing mechanical problems—and there are in the majority of people's bodies—there will be a natural tendency to slump forwards anytime you aren't actively thinking about sitting up straight. Many people these days are, in fact, stuck forwards in their bodies and will spend the majority of their day in a slumped position. If they try to straighten themselves up, it will be short lived because poor alignment and deconditioning will soon have them slumped forwards again. Could it be that a person in a chronically stuck-forwards position is in a state of chronic low confidence? It seems a plausible possibility and something I've noticed people unexpectedly discover when they undergo a structural correction program in my clinic. This unexpected discovery comes in the most lovely of ways as clients and practitioners alike notice a gradual improvement in the client's disposition and attitude towards life.

It's not until they have treatment that they are made aware of what was missing and the dysfunction they had gotten used to and considered normal. Over the years, many clients have reported regaining lost confidence, a feeling of greater freedom, and a stronger ability to handle the stresses of life. It stands to reason that if they are able to have more confidence in their own powers of thinking, the benefits of improved posture on mental state are not only related to the neurology of movement. An improved posture means that there is better breathing, better blood flow, improved mobility, and reduced pain, all of which play their own important role in how we feel moment to moment.

I would argue that the most important way posture impacts health is also the one that's least understood. Thirty years of research by one intrepid Swedish neurosurgeon led to significant breakthroughs in understanding how posture can directly affect the spinal cord and brain by stretching certain spinal soft tissues. I will discuss this little-known aspect of posture in the next chapter because it has potentially far-reaching consequences in terms of the impact of posture on health, but it needs to be understood in the context of how your spine works like a mechanical machine.

It's great to hear about aches, pains, and injuries resolving, but people experience far more benefits than that. Here are a few of the many great changes we hear patients report as their body's alignment and function improves.

UNUSUAL THINGS PATIENTS SAY WHILE UNWINDING

I feel much more confident in myself.

—16-year-old boy who was having a tough time at school

I used to have difficulty buying a shirt to fit me, as my head was so far forward that any shirt collar was rubbing against my ears. Now all shirts now fit me comfortably.

—68-year-old who had major spinal surgery as a child

The arches of my feet have come back after just three sessions of ABC™.

—28-year-old with a lifelong history of flat feet

I ran up the stairs yesterday for the first time in ten years or more. I went back down and tried again, just to make sure.

—50-year-old gardener

I had my suit tailor made to fit my wonky shoulders. That was a waste of money.

—58-year-old CEO

I had all of my shoes built up on the left heel to accommodate for my short leg. Now I need to get them all restored.

—55-year-old businessman

I keep hitting my head on the roof of the car when I get out now!

—40-year-old office worker

My shoulders are now so broad!

—15-year-old rugby player

My feet have grown 1.5 sizes!

—34-year-old doctor

My character has changed so much. I'm not the nervous, anxious person I was before.

—69-year-old retired school teacher

I would normally get really stiff shoulders and a locked up back when I ski. This time, I didn't notice them at all, even after seven full days of skiing!

—50-year-old office worker

I now need to push my head down to see the speedometer on my scooter!

—34-year-old builder

My horse riding coach says that I have become a better rider. The only thing that has changed is getting adjusted!

—55-year-old CEO

My coach commented on the improvement in my running form!

—22-year-old Team GB Sprinter

It looks and feels like I've had a boob lift. I tried on my swimsuit this week, and it looked so different!

—27-year-old chef

I look down on my cousin now, and we have always been the same height!"

—40-year-old fireman

I have been able to get back into tap dancing. I thought I'd never be able to dance again!

—44-year-old dance teacher with chronic foot pain

I saw my neighbour walking around straight for the first time in years. He is normally completely bent over, so that's why I'm here. I had to find out what he was doing!

—75-year-old retired school teacher

I used to have to read for ninety minutes before being able to fall asleep. Now I'm able to drop off in just five minutes.

—29-year-old office worker

I can go lie comfortably on my back and sleep on my back for the first time in 20 years!

—33-year-old Entrepreneur

I keep on bumping my head on the light in the lounge...I never used to reach it!

—38-year-old office worker

CHAPTER 3

Why Posture Goes Wrong

"A healthy person has a thousand wishes, but a sick person has only one"

—*Indian Proverb*

It can be extremely helpful to understand what's going on beneath the surface as body structures go wrong. The fact is, your posture will always bear living witness to what is going on with the overall alignment and health of your joints, which is why I refer to it as the basic measure of structural health. It is the health of the mechanism that powers your machine.

If you remember, the core tenet of the wellness paradigm is that the body has an amazing ability to heal and regulate itself. There is both truth and consequence to this statement. After all, there are only a small number of documented conditions from which no one in the world has been able to heal.

There is, however, an uncomfortable flaw in the premise that the body can heal itself. As remarkable as the intelligent human system is, it is not one hundred percent self-healing. If it were, there would be no need for doctors, and if our posture were ever bent out of shape, we would simply correct it ourselves by stretching. The same approach would work for a broken bone: we would simply contract a muscle, pull the bone back into alignment, and wait for it to heal. Under brief scrutiny, it's easy to acknowledge that even though we are able to fix many things naturally without the help of doctors or chiropractors (even episodes of spinal pain and injury have been known to heal without help), we are not completely self-healing one hundred percent of the time.

In terms of your skeletal and postural health, this means that you are not able to heal every possible problem that may occur within your skeletal framework for one simple yet profound anatomical reason. Perhaps it is a design flaw, or perhaps we haven't fully evolved to meet the demands of modern life inclusive of desks and high-intensity sport, but the fundamental reason that we are not one hundred percent self-healing boils down to a crucial discovery made by Dr. Jesse Jutkowitz, an American chiropractor with a background in mechanical engineering, in the 1980s.

THE STRAIGHT TRUTH

The big discovery that lead to the creation of ABC™ is: bones can go out of alignment in directions from which they cannot self-correct, because we don't have a muscle—or a combination of muscles—that can pull the bone in the direction necessary to return it to its proper position.

Dr. Jutkowitz discovered that bones can go out of alignment in directions from which they cannot self-correct because we don't have a muscle—or a combination of muscles—that can pull the bone in the direction necessary to return it to its proper position. The concept seems so simple, almost too simple, yet it was a missing point of biomechanical understanding for nearly a century before Dr. Jutkowitz was able to work it out.

Bear with me as I explain this because the way that your body deals with problematically misaligned bones has *everything* to do with why you become stuck in a forwards (or slumped) posture, why you keep experiencing the same body problems over and over again regardless of which practitioner you see, and also—most importantly—why your body structurally worsens over time.

Let's make sense of this with the example of a single spinal vertebrae. If one vertebrae were to get stuck out of alignment in the laterally flexed (medical term for sideways bent) position, perhaps due to a fall or an accident, there are muscles in the spine that can contract to pull that vertebrae back into its correct position. If that same vertebrae were to get stuck out of alignment posteriorly (backwards), there are muscles on the front of the body, such as the hip flexors, diaphragm, and others, that could contract in order to bring it back into alignment. Yet, if that same vertebrae were to get stuck in the anterior direction (forwards), there are no muscles at the back of the spine that can contract to pull it backwards. That is the design flaw, the anatomical insufficiency that leaves human bodies vulnerable to structural misalignment (Figure 1A and 1B, Chapter 1).

You can further understand this insufficiency by running your fingers down the back of your spine. Those bony bumps that you feel are called spinous processes, and there is nothing but skin and ligaments attached to the end of each of them. Even if there were a muscle there, where would it attach? It would have to somehow exit your skin and attach to a hook on the wall in order to be able to contract and pull that any one of those spinous processes back into its correct position.

"Hold on a second!" I can already hear you exclaiming. "There *are* muscles down the back of my spine that extend my body backwards." Yes, there are. There are a few spinal extensor muscles that can move several vertebrae at a time into a *generally* backwards extension, but they cannot impart the force necessary to unlock a single vertebrae from a forwards misaligned position. The same biomechanical truth holds for the interspinales muscles (the small muscles that run longitudinally between the individual spinous processes, connecting them together). If they contract, all they do is tilt the vertebra into extension (which does happen as the body attempts to compensate into the next most-balanced alignment); they cannot, however, pull them backwards to their correct position (See Figure 3).

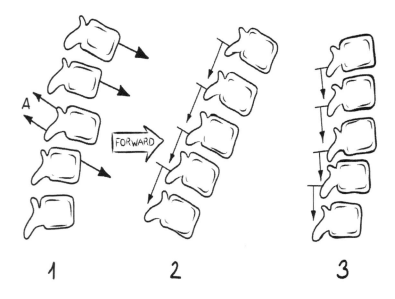

[Figure 3:1] The bone slips forwards and there are no muscles that pull in direction A to retrieve it.

[Figure 3:2] The way muscles actually attach and the direction in which they pull if contracted.

[Figure 3:3] What happens when those muscles contract?

The long and short of it is that if a vertebrae gets stuck in the forwards direction due to external force (there are literally thousands of ways that this can occur, and we'll cover some of them in later chapters), it will stay in that position.

When these vertebrae slip forwards, they may not be able to be pulled back into alignment, but they are still able to move. They are not completely locked up. Muscles can still contract and move the bone, however they don't move the bone correctly. This is an important point to understand because a non-ABC™ healthcare practitioner could examine this area of your spine and discover that the misaligned portion is not especially locked up and, because of that, decide that it is not in need of attention. If you have ever visited a traditional chiropractor or osteopath, you likely understand that these practitioners are, more often than not, searching for the stiff, locked-up regions of your spine and then attempting to get them moving again. As you read on, it will become more clear why this is a mistake.

A final point to understand about this fundamental mechanism in your body is that vertebrae don't just shift forwards; they shift forwards *and* cause a collapse (or fold) in the spine because the shift has caused them to lose most if not all of their leverage ability (see Figure 4).

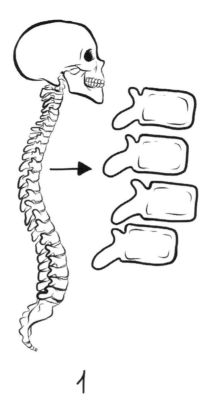

1

[Figure 4:1] What people often think or believe happens if a vertebrae gets misaligned forwards.

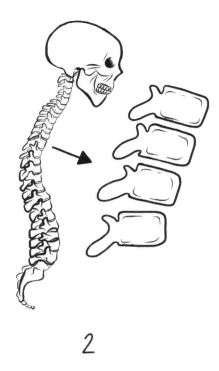

2

[**Figure 4:2**] What actually happens: the vertebrae goes forwards only slightly and loses its leverage, causing a "fold."

Much of the movement in your skeleton occurs through the combination of bones and muscles acting together as levers. For example, when you shake your head back and forth, you use muscles at the front and back of your neck to pivot your skull over your upper neck bones. Standing on your tiptoes is another example; you contract calf muscles to allow you to pivot over your toe joints. When bending your elbow, you contract the front of arm muscle (the biceps) and that force causes the forearm to bend towards your shoulder. These mechanical levers are essential for optimal movement. So much so that if you were to dislocate your shoulder, for example, the lever would be lost such that if you tried to contract your bicep muscle in order to bend your arm, your forearm would simply dangle because the lever had been lost.

A similar mechanism is at play in the spine, albeit to a less obvious degree (because of an inherent backup compensation effect that comes into play). This is why, when your posture is properly corrected using the methods outlined later on, you will find it almost impossible to slump. Truly good posture requires no muscular effort to maintain because the vertebrae and spinal musculature have all of the leverage required to effortlessly maintain you upright against gravity.

This is also why using muscular effort to hold your arms back and lift up your chest is futile for "correcting posture." The stretch may feel good, but it doesn't restore correct anatomical leverage, and therefore, as soon as you get distracted, you will slump again.

The areas where your spine has lost leverage are usually easy to spot. If you take a deep breath in and then let it all out, allowing your body to relax completely, you will feel the areas of your spine where your body wants to collapse forwards. The point at which you notice the most forward curving of your spine is likely where you have a vertebrae slipped into a forwards position and lost some of their leverage. It is also important to note that the section of your spine above that forwards bone is likely to feel quite tight and achy. This is where your body is having to work hard to adapt, or compensate, for the problem bone below.

THE COMPENSATION EFFECT

The loss of bone leverage is only the first in a series of changes that occur in your structure, eventually resulting in poor posture, pain, and diagnosable conditions and syndromes. The forwards-stuck vertebrae is the primary problem and the one that needs to be corrected. If left uncorrected, there will be a predictable cascade of consequences over time.

Let's explore that sequence of events through the example of a scenario whereby a heavy fall onto your buttocks compresses your spine in the middle, locking the T9 bone forwards. As this bone moves forwards, it loses its leverage, which leads to a fold (or compression) in the spine at that point. If your body did nothing to counter this change to its mechanics, your upper body would fall far forwards, and you would lose your balance. Instead, since your brain is continually receiving sensory feedback from your body, it would immediately instruct a change to your overall balance in order to compensate for this misalignment. Your spine would, in effect, be forced to straighten up.

1

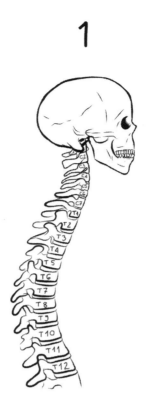

[Figure 5:1] A healthy spine that is correctly aligned.

2

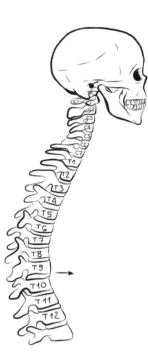

[Figure 5:2] T9 vertebrae gets misaligned (exaggerated for demonstration purposes) and the spine loses its leverage and "folds" at that point.

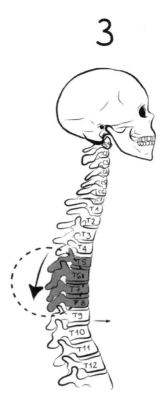

[Figure 5:3] Muscles contract to compensate for the injury, causing tension and eventual symptoms such as back pain.

4

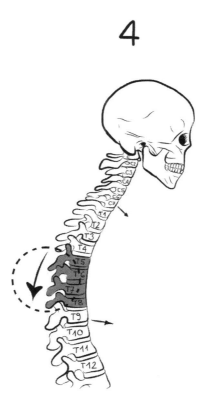

[Figure 5:4] After time or further injury, other bones, such as the C7, also misalign forwards.

5

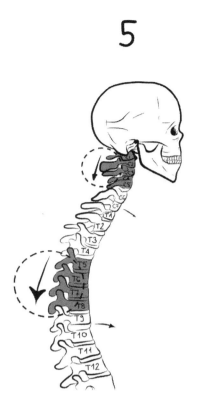

[Figure 5:5] Further compensation in the upper neck and symptoms such as neck pain or headaches.

This compensation requires a continuous muscular effort to maintain stability in the spine, and it's only a matter of time before that effort results in tight and achy muscles or and inflammation and irritation of the joints in your mid-back. As time goes on, another bone in your mid-back, let's say your T4, also gets stuck forwards. There are many reasons why this could happen. Perhaps the compensation for T9 causes you to lean too far backwards, and now something needs to fall forwards in order to balance you. Or, perhaps you experience another trauma that locks your T4 bone forwards.

You now have *two* forwards bones, and you therefore have to compensate even further by leaning back with greater effort, which leads to more compensation tightness in your back. Once again, it is only a matter of time before another bone gets stuck forwards, such as the C7 bone. When the C7 bone moves forwards, the entire head and neck region lose their leverage, and your chin will fall to your chest if you don't make a conscious effort to hold it up. The muscular effort required to raise the chin results in tight muscles and a locking up of joints in the neck. This is how neck pain and headaches correlate with forwards postures. (See Figure 5 above.) Over time, a forward C7 bone, together with the abnormal joint mechanics can cause people to develop a Dowager's hump (a bulbous, usually painless swelling at the base of the neck). A Dowager's hump is not passed down genetically as it's commonly thought to be; it is the result of poor spinal alignment secondary to the primary forwards bone or bones. The early stages of a forwards C7 bone resemble a chicken's neck when, in its most forwards position, and it can be spotted quite easily. People with a forwards C7 bone look like their necks are jutted forward.

One of the important concepts to grasp from this little scenario is that areas that hurt do so because they are under mechanical strain as your body tries to twist, tilt, and lean to compensate for the primary forwards-positioned vertebrae.

The points at which your posture fails are rarely the same points where pain occurs. Interestingly, pain and areas of joint degeneration are almost always found at the points of compensation rather than the points of primary forwards misalignments. These compensation areas become tight and locked into place in order to protect your body and maintain the best possible state of overall balance. This is another example of the innate adaptive intelligence of your body. If your muscles and joints could move more easily out of a tight position, your mechanics would easily worsen, and you'd be in a lot of trouble. Instead, your body twists or tilts to tighten itself up, causing a change in weight-bearing through the joints and altering your body's centre of gravity. Muscles will have to tighten up (and remain tight) in order to protect these newly compensated areas, and this leads to fibrositis and fibrosis (soft tissue inflammation, thickening, and scarring) as well as other tissue strengthening reactions that occur to cope with the extra mechanical load in that region.

There is a dynamic interplay between the primary forwards misalignments, which cannot be self-corrected, and the secondary compensation twisting and tilting that occur as a rebalancing response. Rarely would the pattern be as simple as in the above example. You could have a primary forwards bone paired with compensations, and then get an injury on top of that, which would necessitate its own compensation. The second primary forwards bone-compensation pair could worsen the first, causing the need for another compensation to balance the effect of the first primary forwards-compensation pair. That may, in turn, effect the second primary forwards-compensation pair, requiring another compensation, and on it goes. There is the potential for a highly complicated balancing act to occur, and that is indeed what happens over time.

The conversation gets even more complicated when you include arms and, even more importantly, legs into the equation. Since they are part of the human skeleton, they too can misalign in ways that cannot be self-corrected. They can also tighten and compensate for the greater good of the entire structure. This further explains why some people have more problems when they're sitting down than when they're standing up. When they are standing, the foot, ankle, knee, and hip joints each can be twisted to provide stability against problems in the lower back or pelvis. For this reason, true postural correction requires that the bones of the legs and feet are addressed as well.

Usually, as a person advances in age, he or she will continue to accumulate injuries through their work, sport, or lifestyle (in this case, lifestyle refers to being sedentary or very active; each can cause structural problems). Those changes will most often lead to a gradual increase in structural problems if a person does not receive corrective care for these problems—*real* corrective care, as I have been writing about (an example being the shoulders straightening with no effort) versus what some *call* corrective care that does not truly correct. If a person does not get their alignment corrected over time, either because they choose not to seek out care or seek out corrective care that does not truly correct, the usual outcome is a spine that progressively twists, tightens, and (commonly) falls further forwards. This sort of postural deterioration is easy to spot on people. It is evidenced by unlevel hips, uneven leg lengths, uneven shoulder heights, shoulders that roll forwards, a neck and head that sticks forwards, reduced range of motion in general (usually more noticeable in one direction than the other), and other postural anomalies. If you are thinking that an enormous number of people's bodies fall into that category, you are correct. The main question is, how does that reality adversely affect one's life? Many never know how restricted they have been until their body is corrected with Advanced BioStructural Correction™.

There are many possibilities when it comes to the way the shape of a spine can change over time. The exact posture that a particular body settles into is determined by how that unique body best compensates for its personal series of injuries and misalignments. There is commonly an increase in the mid-back curve, which can make a back look very rounded (known as a hyperkyphosis). Just as common is a straightening of the spine in the thorax (chest); it should instead be just somewhat curved backwards. Neither of these results is good in the longer term, especially because they both compress the chest cavity, reducing one's ability to breathe while compressing the heart. Those whose chest seems to be caved in most often have an overly flat spine in this area.

The lower back may also curve further (known as a hyperlordosis), making it appear as though a person has a pot belly or protruding buttocks. In other cases, a spine degenerates by having its curves flatten, creating what appears to be a very straight back (known as a military spine). Some people's spinal curves actually reverse in direction, causing the mid-back to curve in towards the chest, rather than away from it (known as a thoracic dish), while others will go into rotation, creating a sideways curve (known as scoliosis). Some bodies will lean backwards (known as a sway back), whereas others will lean forwards or sideways from the feet and look like they are tilted off-axis.

There are a great many possible variations, and some people have complex configurations of all the above possibilities. The bottom line is that they all go "wrong" due to the exact same initial *type* of injury—that is, an injury that causes a bone to go out of place in a direction from which the body cannot self-correct because it has no muscle or combination of muscles to pull it in the direction needed to properly reposition it. The area becomes quite unstable, creating imbalances that the body cannot leave unstable and unbalanced. Therefore, the body bends, twists, and rotates those bones in an effort to compensate and stabilise the area. While stabilising that one area, the body moves more off-center and becomes imbalanced in other areas requiring further compensations. It's a balancing act performed by your brain and body to the best of its ability. The way this pattern progresses over time is different for everyone, which explains the huge variety of faulty postures that are possible, and will depend on the nature of their injuries as well as their ongoing lifestyle stresses.

The more problems you accumulate (bones out of place that the body cannot self-correct), the tighter and less robust your body becomes as you work to stabilise and compensate for those bones. This is one of the reasons why people complain about not being able to "get away with" certain activities anymore once they get into their mid-thirties and beyond. The "bouncebackability" of our youth had a lot to do with our bodies' reserve capacity to compensate for problems. The more that your body has to compensate for over the years, the less capacity you have to compensate for new problems until eventually, you wind up chronically injured, and in the worst of cases, unable to stand at all (which does unfortunately happen. I've received several phone calls over the years from patients who were unable to travel; they had become bed-bound as a result of their mechanical problems.)

We discussed the impact of chest function upon heart and lung function in Chapter 3, but another common finding is that symptoms of Chronic Obstructive Pulmonary Disease (COPD) and other breathing issues improve greatly when one's chest shape improves with Advanced BioStructural Correction™. I asked Dr. Jesse Jutkowitz to comment on his experience with correcting the spines of patients who have breathing disorders like COPD, and he commented: "Cases of COPD with blue lips and/or fingers in particular usually pink up within an hour or two of the first treatment, and it gets better from there." To be clear, ABC™ is *not* a treatment for lung or cardiac problems, but as chest function improves, there is often the positive side effect of enhanced function of these important organs. Dr. Jutkowitz is very aware that statements like that can be open to criticism, because they are not typical results seen with traditional approaches to manual therapy. Chest shape and function will not improve unless the proper misalignments are corrected in the right way, together with the meningeal system (which is what ABC™

achieves). He went on to state: "Anyone who criticises me for those statements on chest function has just not been around an Advanced BioStructural Correction™ practice for any amount of time." His challenge to any non-believers is to simply test it out in the real world: "Let them bring a bunch of those people to an Advanced BioStructural Correction™ practitioner before they criticise; that is the only way they will discover the truth." The good news is, the body does not have to stay that way, and in the next chapter we'll look at exactly how the ABC™ methodology addresses and corrects these issues.

By this point, you know more about spinal biomechanics and posture than just about anyone you'll ever meet, but there is another, deeper health consequence to your posture falling forwards that goes way beyond tight muscles and degenerated joints. This additional and important effect that has been demonstrated beyond any reasonable doubt through three decades of clinical neurosurgical research is:

As your posture falls or bends forwards, it stretches your spinal cord, brain stem, brain and nerves coming off of it, like a rubber band.

A failing posture places a stretch tension on your central nervous system. Understanding this is critical to grasping both the symptomatic and health implications of poor spinal alignment. To get a full appreciation of how important this is, we're going to need to take a deeper look into a largely ignored part of your anatomy.

THE DEEP TISSUES

The discovery by Dr. Jesse Jutkowitz that bones go out of alignment in ways that the body cannot self-correct was a major advancement in the field of biomechanics. The understanding of this simple mechanism had a huge impact on our understanding of human bodies as well as our ability to devise treatment strategies to fix them. However, there is much more to the story of why and how the human frame fails. Poor posture has consequences for your spinal cord, nerves, and brain, which can result in a lot of health problems.

To understand this in greater detail, I'd like to introduce you to another poorly understood and often overlooked part of your spinal anatomy—the meninges. The meninges are the protective coverings of your brain and spinal cord. They are made up of three layers that work together as a single functional unit that performs at least two critical jobs. The meninges' first job is to act as an elastic spinal stabiliser, providing internal stability to the motion of your spine and spinal cord. Do you remember those little tourist trinkets of a plastic man held together by elastic tension—when you pushed a button, the elastic went loose and the man flopped down, but when you released the button, he sprang back up? That's a solid analogy for what's going on inside your spine thanks to the elastic tension supplied by the meninges.

The second job of the meninges is to provide the channel through which cerebrospinal fluid circulates. Cerebrospinal fluid (CSF) is thought to act in a manner similar to your body's lymphatic system, helping to cleanse your nervous system of toxins and waste materials. The normal flow of CSF is integral to maintaining a healthy nervous system.

The outer layer of your meninges is a strong, fibrous elastic layer called the Dura Mater. The middle layer is known as the Arachnoid Mater (so called because it looks like a spider web), and the inner layer that attaches to the outer surface of the spinal cord is called the Pia Mater. There endeth the detailed anatomy lesson!

When your spine bends forwards, the meninges (as well as your spinal cord) are pulled over the back of the inside of the vertebral bodies, stretching them tighter. It's a bit like when you tuck your shirt in and then bend forwards, causing it to become stretched along the length of your back. Your brain, brainstem, and nerves also get stretched, albeit indirectly, as a consequence of the same mechanism, because it is all connected in one functional system.

In a normal, healthy spine there is actually quite a lot of stretch in the spinal cord. Dr. Alf Breig was the neurosurgeon who carried out those three decades of research that I mentioned previously. He discovered that as your head moves from full extension to full flexion, the spinal cord stretches at least 3cm. Far from being in a constantly static state, the spinal cord and nerves move in a dynamic manner, which means that they will be forced to adapt to changes in your posture, placing even greater importance upon your alignment.

Your meninges are a tube, and because of the way its fibres interweave they respond in interesting ways to spinal movement. When stretched, the diameter of the tube narrows, squeezing the spinal cord, brainstem and brain. The effect is similar to a Chinese handcuff—you know, those woven tubes that you place around your fingers, and when you try and pull them apart, they clamp down. When the spine is optimally aligned in the upright position, there is no stretch on the meninges and zero mechanical pressure on the nervous system. In this relaxed state, function is normal and optimal neurologically. When a normal, uninjured spine bends forwards, because of the stretching effect on the meninges there will be a narrowing of the meninges with a non-problematic squeezing effect on the brain and spinal cord. If, however, a spine gets misaligned and one's posture distorts in any of the many ways mentioned earlier in the chapter, there can be a stretch of the meninges beyond the normal range. This can cause a much more significant traction and compression effect on the spinal cord and nerves that branch off of it, leading to many potential health problems. In some people, the stretch goes down the body, resulting in various problems in breathing as well as affecting lower-back nerves, creating back and leg pain. In others, the stretch goes up the body, affecting their arms, neck, and even into the head, causing brain fog or the inability to think well.

The abnormal mechanical stress on the meninges causes them to become irritated and worn, ultimately causing a scarring reaction whereby the tissues are drawn together in an attempt to adapt and heal. The effect is similar to the scar you would create were you to repetitively stretch, rub, and compress your skin beyond its normal range of tolerance.

When the meninges are overstretched and scarred, they can also become fixed to the spinal column, which can have the effect of locking spinal misalignments together in a mechanical pattern that *cannot be changed* as long at these adhesions remain. This is important to understand because it explains why many traditional manual and manipulative therapies, including rehabilitative exercises, fail to properly and consistently correct posture. Any changes that *are* made are soon lost as the internal mechanical tension from these meningeal adhesions forces the spine back into a misaligned position.

If you have been back and forth to many practitioners for the same problem—one that only gets better for a short time before returning—you now understand one of the key reasons why that happens. Unless meninges are addressed and helped to relax and heal, the same mechanical pattern has no choice but to remain. Believe it or not, it's helping your body to remain stable. Uncorrected meningeal adhesions are one of the main reasons why it's impossible to correct your own alignment to any significant degree with exercise alone, including the use of spinal traction devices, wedges, or straps commonly sold online. They may make you feel better temporarily, but once you stop using them, your body will, sooner or later, change back into a distorted and dysfunctional posture.

This phenomenon also explains why people get stuck in the hard kyphotic position (where the spine is stuck in the forwards position with an exaggerated mid-back curve), unable to touch their head to the floor when they lie on their back. They are literally locked into place by meningeal adhesions. No amount of home stretching, massage, or traditional manipulation will have any lasting impact. These individuals often have big problems with sleep apnea and snoring. The reasons for that once again boil down to basic anatomy.

Your meninges wrap around your brain and spinal cord like a sleeping bag, and throughout most of the spine they hang freely, only loosely attached to the spinal column by thin ligaments known as dentate ligaments. There are, however, a few points where the meninges anchor and attach firmly to your structure: the coccyx (tail bone), the second cervical vertebra, and at multiple points inside the skull, including the back of the bones that make up your face. These points of meningeal tethering in your skull are crucial to how your body works mechanically.

To better understand the impact that meningeal adhesions have on your own body's function, you can perform a simple experiment.

EXPERIMENT

Stand upright in your normal, relaxed posture. Take a deep breath in through your nose. Notice the quality of your breath, the depth, the amount of movement, and the ease of movement in your rib cage as well as the ease with which air passes in and out of your nose.

Now, take your fist and place it under your chin, gently lifting your chin upwards by about one centimetre allowing your neck and back muscles to relax completely (this experiment has even better results if someone else supports your chin so that you can relax more completely). Take another breath in through your nose and notice how it feels. The vast majority of people who do this experiment will notice an improvement in their breathing, with air passing more easily through the nasal passages and their rib cage able to expand further and with less effort. If you do not notice the difference, take your hand away from your chin and breathe again. You will likely notice that it feels more restricted.

How could this simple trick improve your breathing? Placing your hand under your chin and putting your neck into a slight extension has the effect of taking tension *out* of the meningeal system. Since the meninges are attached to the bones of your face, including the bones that make up the nasal passages, there is now less mechanical restriction to your airways, making it easier to breathe.

There is a two-way relationship between the spine and the cranial system (the skull bones and connective tissues inside the head), because they are linked together via the meninges and, even though many treat them separately, they are really not separate systems. If the spine misaligns, the meningeal tension created can distort the cranial system, adversely affecting it and creating problems such as breathing restrictions, blocked sinuses, or headaches. In fact, the problems created can be related to a great deal of problems body-wide, not just locally. On the other hand, if you suffered any past head or facial trauma, from surgery, dentistry, accidents or injuries, the cranial bones can become misaligned, leading to tension on the meningeal system and an adverse effect on the alignment of the rest of the spine and body. That is why a part of the ABC™ method involves cranial work. We call it ABC Endonasal Cranial Correction™, and it essentially involves gentle manipulation of the cranial bones by safely inflating small balloons inside the patient's sinus cavities. The results from this aspect of ABC™ treatment can be remarkable with respect to any pain the patient is experiencing, but people are often pleasantly surprised to also see positive changes in how their face looks when comparing their before and after pictures. It is quite usual to notice improved symmetry and a reduction in wrinkles as a result of restoring structural alignment to the skull.

UNWINDING STORIES

I haven't slept in the same room as my wife for years because my snoring would wake her up. After my first ABC Endonasal Cranial Correction™ treatment, my snoring stopped and I have been allowed back in the bedroom.

—Dave, 42, Builder

I couldn't believe the before and after photos. It was clear that my eyes appeared to level out, which seemed unbelievable. But when I got home, I looked back over old photos of me and, sure enough, you can clearly see that my left eye has always been lower than me right. Not anymore!

—Ross, 53, IT Consultant

It was amazing. The intense headache behind my eye lifted almost straight away after the cranial correction. Normally those bad headaches stay with me for days

—Susanne, 44, Medical Doctor

I've been able to breathe clearly through my nose again!

—48-year-old office worker with a lifelong history of nose breathing difficulties

My nose is straight again!

—*Stuart, 26, Dance Teacher*

The meningeal system is crucial to the way in which your spine moves. It is so often ignored or inadequately addressed by spinal health practitioners. Correctly treating this meningeal system to release the points of scarring or adhesion is crucial to restoring proper alignment and motion to the body. However, it is still only one part of a much bigger system—your overall body structure. It is important to know that you are not made up of simply a neck, back, and pelvis. You are a whole system, made up of a complete spine, cranium, jaw, pelvis, meninges, arms, and legs, which all work together as a singular synchronised functioning unit (See Figure 6). A traumatic injury or problem in one area automatically leads to an abnormal reaction throughout the entire structural system. Understanding this helps explain why people so often get stuck into a fixed pattern of poor posture or injury which they cannot get out of. This postural pattern is really just an intelligent adaptation of their body to the main problem (or a series of layered problems) that cannot be self-corrected. The next best option that your body has is to lock you up in a tension pattern that allows you to function as best as you can, in a "new normal" so to speak, given the problems your body has taken on. The fact that your whole skeletal frame works together in synchronous function also explains why not everyone gets better with traditional methods of treatment. Therapy is often only applied to the area that hurts, and the interrelated areas of the structure—which likely also have misalignments related to the presenting problem—are ignored. Unless the entire body's mechanical structure is examined and treated appropriately where problems are found, there will be a tendency for failed treatments or a return of pain at a later date.

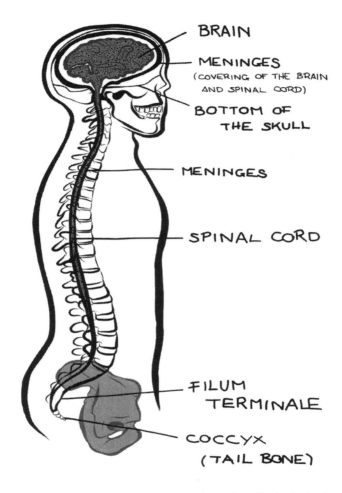

BRAIN

MENINGES
(COVERING OF THE BRAIN
AND SPINAL CORD)

BOTTOM OF
THE SKULL

MENINGES

SPINAL CORD

FILUM
TERMINALE

COCCYX
(TAIL BONE)

[Figure 6] The normal spinal-meningeal relationship: The brain, brainstem, spinal column, pelvis and meninges act as a singular synchronised functioning unit. Abnormal or traumatic action within one area automatically and synchronously results in abnormal reaction throughout the entire unit. This often results in an abnormal and fixed structural stress holding pattern, or posture.

THE NEUROSURGEONS WHO FIGURED THIS OUT

Much of what we now understand about the meningeal system and the negative neurological effects that result from it being physically stretched were initially discovered by Swedish neurosurgeon Dr. Alf Breig. Throughout the 1960s, '70s, and '80s, he diligently researched the negative health impacts of what he termed "adverse mechanical tension of the nervous system." He was the first to recognise the problems associated with stretched and scarred meninges and the way they put pressure on parts of the brain and spinal cord.

Dr. Breig developed a pioneering neurosurgical method to help his patients. This method involved surgically attaching a ribbon to the base of a patient's skull, then running it under the skin and securing the other end to the thoracic spine (mid-back). The aim behind this method was to hold a patient's head in slight extension and take the mechanical tension out of hyper-elongated meninges and the central nervous system (a more advanced approach to the breathing experiment you tried earlier in this chapter). He discovered that this produced a profound reduction of neurological symptoms in his patients. They were not simple cases either; we are talking about patients with serious conditions like multiple sclerosis, amyotrophic lateral sclerosis (ALS), spinal fractures, and other serious spinal cord injuries.

After thirty years of clinical research and application of these principles, Dr. Breig stated in his final textbook, *Skull Traction and Cervical Cord Injury,* that Multiple Sclerosis, ALS, and other diseases of that type are probably not diseases at all. They are different manifestations of adverse mechanical tension within the central nervous system, caused by various sorts of mechanical pathologies in the spine, forcing the spine into flexion and stretching the spinal cord and brainstem. That was quite a significant and challenging statement to make, especially in the age of pharmaceutical medicine, when the treatment of choice is usually medication.

Another groundbreaking paper was published in 2000 (and again in 2004) by neurosurgeon Dr. Shokei Yamada, who developed a surgery to treat something known as Tethered Cord Syndrome. This is a complex condition whereby the spinal cord is stretched to a significant enough degree that some of the nerves stop working altogether. It presents in a way similar to sciatica with back and leg pain, but the condition is generally more severe and harder to treat due to the mechanical effect of tight meninges. His approach to reduce pressure on the central nervous system was to surgically cut the scars and fibrous tissues of the meninges at the base of the spine in a region of the lower back known as the filum terminale. This method also created excellent results for patients, with virtually all patients experiencing improvements in neurological function. Up to ninety-five percent of patients experienced complete relief from severe back pain.

The work of both Dr. Breig and Dr. Yamada was instrumental in understanding the role of the meningeal system on neurological and structural health. The important take-home message is not that you need to have neurosurgery to correct your body (unless your condition progresses incredibly severely), but rather, we now know how important a role these structures play, and the huge impact that meningeal scarring, adhesion, and tension can have upon the workings of the nervous system.

The results created by these two amazing surgeons are remarkable, but they came at a cost. Dr Breig's patients had dramatic reduction in symptoms, but also a permanent reduction in their range of motion. Dr Yamada's patients had excellent results, but their meningeal adhesions above the lower back were not corrected and continued to drag on their spine, albeit to a lesser extent. Also, one doesn't know whether the robustness of their body was impacted over time. For the patients whom these surgeons treated, the tradeoff was likely worth it; they are serious pathologies that had progressed quite far down the road of dysfunction. In both scenarios, the underlying cause of the patients' meningeal tension and spinal cord stretching was not addressed. All that was treated were the downstream, late-stage effects. Nonetheless, their treatments provided a valuable service, rushing in with their axes and firehoses and saving significant additional stress to as well as possible loss of the metaphorical house's life.

What if there were a way to address the underlying mechanical cause of spinal cord tension? What if the subsidence causing the mechanical pressure could be reversed, and the structure stabilised? What if it were possible to rebuild a spine back to normal, relaxed alignment wherein the mechanical pressure were taken out of the whole system, preserving the long-term function of the body?

Good news: there is. And it's exactly what we'll dive into in the next chapter.

RICARDA'S UNWINDING STORY

Student, 14

Before I started my treatment at SpineCentral, I suffered with severe neck pain and had very bad posture due to my scoliosis. My posture was visibly slanted, and I leaned forward and to my left with my right shoulder sticking up and my rib cage pointing out. My dad used to say that I ran "like a duck." However, after I started my ABC™

treatment with Richard and his team, my posture greatly improved within weeks. As they corrected my alignment, I began to stand a lot straighter and my neck pain gradually went away. The spine central team isn't just amazing in what they do, they are also all really lovely and interesting people. I thank them very much for helping to fix my spine. My dad and I travel a great distance to get the treatment, which has certainly helped. We are very pleased.

CHAPTER 4

The Primary Domino Effect

"There is a vast difference between treating the effects and
adjusting the cause"

—*D.D. Palmer*

We covered a lot of ground in the previous chapter, and you learned that there is a primary domino when it comes to structural problems in the body. When the primary domino falls, a chain reaction begins a cascade of consequences through the entire skeleton. There are many ways to create these primary forwards-stuck bones in your body. Let's explore a few of the more common ones:

A Traumatic Fall

Falling onto your back or buttocks as well as any heavy impact anywhere on your body has the potential to push bones out of alignment.

Prolonged Poor Postures

Habitual slumping at work or at home due to poor ergonomics or the wrong choice of chair can, over time, put forces on your back that have the same consequences.

Excessive Stretching

Extreme or repetitive forward bending, as is commonly done in disciplines like yoga and Pilates, can also lock you forwards. Back-bending can have the same effect, because when you lean back, there is a cantilever effect that simultaneously produces a strong forwards force, usually in the lower back.

Contact Sports

There are many of these wherein accidents can happen, such as football, rugby, or martial arts.

A Car Crash

When the head whips forwards there can be a strong forward pull onto the bones, which locks them in the forwards position. Equally, when the mid-back slams backwards into the seat, bones can get stuck forwards from that reactive force as well. In my experience, failure to address forwards-stuck bones from a whiplash injury is one of the main reasons symptoms commonly persist in patients, sometimes for years, until full spine alignment is correctly restored.

Remember, your body cannot fix forwards-stuck bones, regardless of how they are caused, for the simple anatomical reason that you don't have any muscles that can contract to do the job. Instead, your body will tilt and twist to lock up multiple bones in an effort to compensate for and stabilise the injured area. The devil is in the details here. The forwards-stuck bone loses leverage but *does not lock up completely* (that's a really important point). The twisting and tilting forces of the compensation effort cause a shift in the balance of your posture as a new dynamic tension spreads throughout your whole body. It's like rotating a Rubik's Cube; changing the pattern on one side affects all six sides of the cube. As time goes on, the more changes that are introduced into the system, the further you stray from the perfect pattern, the more complex the problem becomes, and the greater likelihood that you will experience pain or injury.

There is a simple way to experience this dynamic connection between all the parts of your body in real time, through the following anatomy experiment:

EXPERIMENT

Sit relaxed in a chair and turn your head from left to right. Notice how far you can comfortably turn it and what sort of tension you feel in the movement. Now, scrunch up the toes on both of your feet tightly, hold them in the scrunched position, and redo the test. Depending upon your unique body alignment, you will find that you can turn your head more one way or less the other way, more both ways, or less both ways. Also pay attention to how your breathing changes before you scrunch up your toes and after. It might increase or decrease in depth. The key point is that you will notice a subtle change in neck movement or breathing depth just by changing the alignment of your toes!

I tested this on my own body as I sat down to write this chapter, and I found that I can look further in both directions when my toes are scrunched up. From a biomechanical perspective, what is happening is that the increased joint, muscle, and fascial tension created in my feet when I scrunch my toes spreads all the way up my body, providing enhanced stability for bone(s) stuck in positions that cannot be self-corrected somewhere. The overall effect is improved mechanical movement and support all the way up to my neck. My ability to breathe also improves as I scrunch my toes. You may find the opposite scenario to be true for your body. It depends upon how your body is compensating for its mechanical problems.

THE GRADUAL BUILD-UP OF STRUCTURAL PROBLEMS

If you were to have only one primary forwards bone, you probably wouldn't even notice the tightening of your structure as it performs its rebalancing act. This is typically what happens early in life. A trained eye can pick up the subtle postural clues of a body falling and twisting, but the person who is living in that body will most likely not notice the changes.

If you have an accident and add another primary forwards bone into the mix, you will have two major problems with possibly several compensation patterns, adding more twisting stress into your body. At this point, you might start to notice that you're a bit stiffer than you used to be. Perhaps your breathing is a bit more restricted, but you only notice that restriction if you play sports or are in a rush. On the whole, you still live life with excellent function.

Throw in a few more years of sitting at a desk for eight hours per day and a skiing accident that caused you to roll down that black diamond run. Now, your shoulders, neck, and upper back feel stiff, especially towards the end of the day. You notice that your left knee tightens up and sometimes hurts after long runs. You've had two episodes in the last year where your lower back locked up and left you in agony for a few days. Most mornings, you wake up feeling stiff, and it takes several minutes to several hours to loosen up and get going. Long walks or long periods of standing—in fact long periods time spent doing *anything*—are becoming a problem. Your body seems to complain a lot more than it used to, and you are beginning to "feel your age." You are secretly wondering what sort of shape your body will be in by the time you reach your seventies!

There are lots of possible signs and symptoms that can occur as your structure comes under increasing mechanical tension. You may notice that your neck doesn't turn as easily as it used to, making it more difficult to look behind you as you reverse your car or change lanes in traffic. Perhaps you notice that your back doesn't twist as well in one direction, and it's easy to cross your legs one way, but feels strange to cross them the opposite way. You may notice that you don't recover from exercise with the same speed that you used to. Muscular soreness seems to be more intense and longer-lasting after your workouts. You may experience niggling injuries or find that you are getting injured more frequently. Your back might ache on long bike rides, runs, or swims. Another common complaint is feeling "locked up" after working out in the gym.

The result of increased mechanical tension can manifest in symptoms such as headaches, jaw pain and clicking, brain fog, irritability, body tension, aches and pains, sciatica, sports injuries, tiredness, muscular pains and tenderness, and even various organ system issues. The exact symptom (or symptoms) will depend on your unique structural tension pattern and how you have stressed it over the years. It's when the body reaches this symptomatic stage that most people will start seeking help, either by calling a professional or trying to help themselves through various stretching or strengthening exercises learned from YouTube. After all, if it feels tight, you should stretch it out. Right?

Wrong! When you fully grasp the underlying mechanism of how body structures go wrong, you recognize that the tightness is there for a reason. It is part of your body's attempt to stabilise itself.

SPRING LOADED AND WOUND UP TIGHT

Imagine your body as a giant metal coil. If you twist the coil, a kink will appear, and that section of the coil that used to be loose will now be under tension. If you keep twisting, you will soon get more kinks in the coil. If you continue to stretch, several kinks may twist together and form a larger kink and so on into a progressively tighter pattern with all kinds of strange—but necessary—new forces running through the coil. This is quite similar to what happens in your spine. The vertebrae twist and shift, and elastic tension is created from the meningeal system inside the spine getting stretched forwards and then scarring, shrinking, and locking you into place. Further mechanical tension is created from the compensation pattern, locking up bones and tightening the lines of tough fascia which run head to toe throughout your body. The points in your structure where the mechanical tension and locking are greatest are the exact points at which you will experience the greatest symptoms. Eventually, given enough years or mechanical stress (perhaps accelerated through participating in intensive sports or a working a manual labour job, or even from being overly sedentary), these are the same points at which degenerative arthritis will occur. A joint that isn't moving correctly and is under increased mechanical demands will cause greater stress to be placed on the cartilage, allowing for more frequent injuries, inflammation, and ongoing repair. The result is early degeneration.

There are other nutritional factors that can increase the speed and severity with which joint degeneration progresses. Smoking, nutritional deficiencies, and excessive sugar consumption are known contributing factors. You should know, however, that excessive biomechanical loading of the joints is the key factor at play in most cases of joint degeneration, which is also known as osteoarthritis.

JOINTS OUT OF ALIGNMENT THAT YOU CAN FIX?

At this point, you may have an important question weighing on your mind: What happens to the joints that are out of alignment in a direction whereby the body *can* fix them (because the joint *does* have muscles that can contract to pull it back to alignment), but it doesn't, and the joint remains stuck. This is a scenario that would logically have to occur in the body to explain the wide variation of postures and alignments seen in different people.

At first glance, this scenario could appear to reveal a hole in the theories behind structural correction, but with a bit of common sense the point is easily understood. These types of misalignment cannot be unlocked by the body because they are part of a compensation pattern that is actually *making you stable.* This means that if the body were to fix the issue, you would mechanically worsen. Nonetheless, people do go against the wisdom of their body with methods of self-manipulation, such as lying on their back and twisting their knees to the side to "click" their tension away. Or, forcefully squeezing their shoulders backwards to "pop" the joints in their mid-back. My favourite method I hear people talk about: "getting the wife to walk on my back." Even Homer Simpson figured out that if he pushed people backwards over a bin, they felt better afterwards. By the way, if you haven't seen this clip, it's well worth the three minutes it will take you to find and watch it on YouTube. Homer beautifully sums up the challenges and misunderstandings within the world of manual therapies, and he doesn't make chiropractic profession look very good in the process!

People almost always report feeling much better after doing this sort of self-manipulation. The issue, however, is that they couldn't possibly have corrected a forwards bone by bringing it backwards. The only thing they could have done is forcibly release a compensation pattern. This is exactly what happens, of course, because the only reason the joint was bothering them was because it was locked up and under tension in order to compensate for a loss of leverage somewhere else in the body. Releasing that tension will nearly always feel good, but that does not mean that it actually did you any good mechanically, or that you should do it. If you do, your body will have to immediately get back to re-creating the compensation pattern, which is why you generally find that a few hours later, the tension returns to the same spot. If you were to check a person's posture immediately after these sorts of self-manipulation moves, you would find their mechanics to be worse; there will be a fold somewhere as they breathe out, and the breath quality will be reduced.

THE PROBLEM WITH MOST FORMS OF MANIPULATIVE THERAPY

The examples given above include crude forms of self-manipulation that have been around for at least 3,000 years. Trying to manipulate your own bones or joints for quick relief has limited effectiveness because you can only use long, broad levers and cannot isolate any specific bone (let alone the ones that are stuck forwards).

This is where most manipulative arts come in to play. There are many throughout the world, and they typically fall into three main professions: chiropractic, osteopathy, and physiotherapy. Interestingly, physiotherapy never used to be about spinal manipulation. It wasn't until recently that its effectiveness in terms of pain relief started to become more widely known, and physiotherapists began learning some techniques to move bones.

Most chiropractors, including myself, sometimes get twitchy about using the terms *manipulation* and *adjustment* interchangeably. They are often confused, and they are not the same thing. There is a big difference between these two approaches in terms of both the art of delivery and the intended outcome of the procedure. These differences are important to understand, so I will attempt to explain them as well as the reasons why neither method, when applied within any of the traditional approaches, can truly correct your body mechanics to the point that your posture will stand tall without any effort.

A manipulation is typically a bigger movement and force performed over a section of the spine using a long lever in an attempt to mobilise the region of joints. There are often a few "cracks" heard during a manipulation, which are really just the after-effect of nitric oxide gas expanding within the joint capsules. An adjustment, on the other hand, is usually a lighter, more specific force aimed at restoring the alignment and motion of a single bone. It is typically a faster, crisper, and more skilled procedure with a more detailed examination process conducted before the adjustment is delivered in order to work out what's gone wrong to begin with and what needs to happen to correct that specific bone's alignment. This more detailed and specific approach typically creates better outcomes for patients.

The subtle nuances between a manipulation and an adjustment are important because the art and science of the profession are wrapped up in them. When push comes to shove, however, both adjusting and manipulating are about moving bones. Patients often wonder how a practitioner determines which bones to move. The answer nearly always lies in checking the body to assess which bones are locked up where there is pain. The issue with this approach is that, as mentioned earlier, the bones that are locked up and tender are part of a compensation pattern, and they are not the primary bones to be corrected.

Not only are the bones involved in the compensation found where it hurts the most, they are also often surrounded by tight muscles wherein you are likely to find the nerves most stretched and pressurised. It's also where X-rays and MRIs are likely to reveal most of the long-term degenerative effects. A skilled traditional chiropractor or osteopath trained in the art of tracking down these problems will invariably expertly find and correct these stuck bones, which are actually compensations that should, arguably, be left alone.

There are only a few possible outcomes when this traditional approach is used to adjust or manipulate the bones that are most stuck. Nearly always, the patient will feel better after an adjustment, especially if there was a specific adjustment done to the bone that was out of alignment at the peak point of compensation. This in itself is not necessarily a "bad" intervention, and in fact it is often a good thing to do from the perspective of reducing pain quickly and allowing a patient to get back to living his life. The problem is that the body will immediately begin recreating the compensation pattern, sometimes even by the time the patient has walked to the reception desk to pay. Oftentimes, however, it will take days to weeks to recreate the compensation pattern to the point that one will notice symptoms again. Either way, the patient will end up complaining about the same symptom returning. Does that sound familiar? Do you find that the same aches, pains, and problems frustratingly return, even after you have been manipulated or adjusted? Beneath the surface, your body has simply recreated the compensation pattern that was temporarily wiped out by the practitioner or yourself (with self-manipulation).

Another possible outcome of releasing compensations is that the body shifts the tension pattern elsewhere, causing new symptoms. Perhaps you went to the practitioner with back pain that resolved, but the next day you woke up with a stiff neck. Although rare, there could also be an immediate and significant worsening of symptoms if an important compensation is removed, leaving an unstable section of the spine unsupported. Eventually, the body will rebuild the compensation and again find stability, but this sort of problem can and should be avoided.

THE TIGHTNESS IS THE SOLUTION, NOT THE PROBLEM

The temptation to stretch, massage, or foam roll away your tension should also be pursued with caution because, once again, it is done with the assumption that the pain or tightness is the problem. It's not; it's part of the solution. It seems that most of the patients who have visited my office over the years have felt compelled to stretch. They often want to know which stretches to do to help their bodies, and they're quite surprised when I tell them that they don't need to stretch in order to get better. In fact, I usually discourage them from doing so. If you forcibly release tight tissues, you risk worsening your mechanics. You may improve the length of muscles or the mobility of joints in one area of your body, but that will adversely affect the function of your body somewhere else. You can spot this sort of bittersweet effect by testing your breathing and postural stability before and after any stretching, mobilising, or foam rolling, using the structural self-assessment technique provided in Chapter 1.

I'm not sure where or how the myth that stretching is the solution began, but it is well and truly alive, and the rise in popularity of yoga has only fanned the flames and added to the misunderstanding. There is nothing inherently wrong with yoga, Pilates, or any similar activity. In fact, they can be beneficial practices to integrate body and mind, release stress, and improve your fitness. But, you should also appreciate that they are *balanced disciplines for balanced bodies*. If you are walking around in a highly torqued and compensated state, you will feel awfully stiff. It is forgivable to think that the solution could be found by stretching away the tightness, but now that you understand why these muscles get tight in the first place, it no longer makes sense to keep undoing your brains attempts to stabilise your body.

Some people like to work on stretching to lengthen their muscles or their mobility to improve a joint's range of motion. Sometimes, it can help with achieving certain favourable positions in sports such as ballet or martial arts. The risks of pursuing greater flexibility, however, should be understood and appreciated. Interestingly, what has been noted in the work of hundreds of ABC™ practitioners around the world is that when patients adopt a routine of regular stretching, it does not speed up their journey through structural correction. Whilst the impact can sometimes be very minimal (if done with due care and attention), it can also have the negative impact on slowing down, hampering, or completely impeding the process of structural correction.

At best, stretching is a neutral activity. It usually feels quite good to stretch, but at the same time you know that the muscle or muscles will likely be tight again by the next day, perhaps even by the end of the current day. If you keep up your routine, you will eventually make progress and feel as though you are becoming more limber. But, what happens if you stop your daily practice? It won't take long for your body to build up the tightness again. Usually, within a week or two you will be back to where you were when you first started your stretching practice.

The worst-case scenario (which does happen, albeit rarely), is that people make themselves significantly worse off symptomatically by engaging in a stretching practice. This happens when one's body falls further forwards into an injury because a tension that was helping your stability is released. Or, because one manages to push something forwards in the process of stretching. In fact, there is a fair bit of research these days showing that stretching actually increases the rate of injury among athletes, especially if done before the sport as part of the warm up.[28,29,30] This should be no surprise now that you understand what is going on mechanically in your body when you stretch.

You might find it interesting that yoga and Pilates teachers' bodies are some of the most challenging that I've worked with over the years, for the simple reason that they continue to create problems through their training. It is very challenging to help these people get to a good enough place mechanically that they do not require some form of ongoing treatment. Equally, the most chronically injured athletes I've seen are quite twisted and forwards in their structure, which explains why they feel a constant need to be stretching.

If you love participating in yoga, Pilates, and similar practices, you can chose to keep participating in them, but it is important to pay close attention to the ways in which you are moving and putting force on your body, taking care not to force any stretch and keeping perfect form throughout (much more on this topic in Chapter 9). Once again, test your own posture to see if you are improving or worsening mechanically as you progress in your practice. If you are an athlete, it is better not to stretch before you train or compete, and instead focus on full body functional movements to get warmed up.

Massage fits into the same camp as stretching, unfortunately, but it can be even more problematic mechanically. Not only does it release compensation tension, it is usually performed with the patient lying face-down with an often heavy pressure pushing from backwards to forwards, creating new forwards stuck bones or worsening existing ones. The combination can worsen one's mechanics, and it is often easy to tell that this has happened when you stand up after the massage because you have a light-headed, woozy feeling, which people mistakenly believe is the result of being relaxed. In reality, it is much more likely to be the result of increased brain stem and spinal cord tension from a posture that has been pushed forwards.

Don't be too concerned at this point if you participate in any or all of the above modalities and love them because you feel better or looser afterwards. If you get your body mechanics treated correctly by an ABC™ practitioner, you will find that your body rarely—if ever—develops tension or feels the need to be massaged or stretched in the first place. When your body mechanically improves to a significant enough degree, the usual feedback is that people no longer get the same enjoyment factor out of stretching or massages and eventually notice that these activities are, in fact, bothersome.

There are many different stretches, disciplines, and body conditioning practices. There are also many different types of chiropractors, osteopaths, and physiotherapists with varying techniques and approaches. Each of these approaches will provide relief for a certain number of people, helping them to feel better. There are lots of ways to remove tension from the system and improve it symptomatically. There are also many theories on what is going on beneath the surface when body treatment or training is carried out.

However, if your results are going to be consistent and predictable, you *must* improve the foundational alignment and mechanical function, not just treat the symptoms—even if you're doing so in safe and natural ways. Remember, the paradigm that drives the questions is what determines the results. If you focus on rebuilding the foundation so that the whole building can be strong and healthy, you will get different results than if you continue only to hammer down the squeaky floor boards once a month. Thankfully, the ABC™ method offers a consistent and predictable option to correct your body so that you can rebuild your structural foundation.

THE NEW POSTURE CORRECTION METHOD

Much of what you have now learned about the way your spine misaligns and adapts was discovered by Dr. Jutkowitz. Unsatisfied with the inconsistent results of traditional chiropractic techniques, he employed his background in mechanical engineering to set about attempting to discover the mechanical reason why human structures fail. Through his extensive research, which included the mathematical analysis of sitting and standing both pre- and post-X-rays, he was able to understand the three-dimensional mechanics of the way the human spine misaligns, and how this misalignment affects all the systems of the body. He is famous for stating that "all health problems, excluding cancer, infections, fractures, diabetes, and the likes are easily understood with the knowledge that they are effects of structural problems that the body cannot self-correct." This holds true even on the molecular level, where much of the way a cell behaves comes down to its 3D structure in space.

Dr. Jutkowitz describes Advanced BioStructural Correction™ as "a protocol to both find and correct things in the body that have gone out of place in directions that the body cannot self-correct." This method is different from other adjustment methods in the sense that it *only* attempts to correct problems that the body cannot fix by itself.

In particular, this includes two main issues, both of which you're familiar with by this point: meningeal scars and forwards-stuck bones (Primary BioStructural Pathologies, or Primaries for short, in ABC™ terminology). The ABC™ method is the only adjusting technique available that gets consistent and predictable positive effects—precisely because it addresses both of those issues. Interestingly, it does this with a style of adjusting that is almost precisely opposite that of traditional methods. Rather than putting a force on the spine from a backwards-to-forwards direction, ABC™

adjustments aim to "lift" bones back into position with either standing- or rolling-type adjustments that apply forwards-to-backwards pressures to the spine. ABC™ is also different in that it is a full-body system that also address misalignments of the ribs, pelvis, knees, feet, ankles, and cranial bones with specific adjustment techniques. A typical treatment session scans the body from head to toe for bones that are misaligned in positions from which the body cannot correct and adjusts them back into their correct positions.

After one session of ABC™, your body's ability to hold itself upright immediately improves because the mechanical leverage of your spine has been restored as the primaries are corrected, and the tight meningeal scars have been reduced so that they don't pull you back into the same posture as before.

Once these primary misalignments have been addressed, your spine is able to release the compensation patterns, a process that can take some time but creates a noticeable reduction in pain, tension, and stiffness, even after the first session. When people first hear this, it often sounds like too much to promise or as though, somehow, it's mere hype. I thought so too—until I experienced the results on myself and then witnessed them play out in thousands of patients. Before anyone is adjusted in my office or in the office of any ABC™ practitioner around the world, a posture picture is taken after the patient is given these exact instructions: "Breathe in, breathe out, let your body slump and relax." At the beginning of treatment, most people have a significant fold or collapse in their posture with their head dropping down, their back and shoulders rounding, and a forwards (as well as often a sideways) tilt to their body.

Even after the first adjustments, when the pictures are retaken after the patient is given the same instructions to breathe in, breathe out, and relax, we see an immediate improvement in the patient's posture. Patients can feel this improvement as well. There is no advice given to hold their body in any specific way; in fact, the exact opposite instruction is given. Patients are instructed to let go of their muscular tension. No rehabilitation of muscles is carried out during a treatment session. The only reason that the patient is standing better by the end is that his alignment been improved by the ABC™ treatment process, and he has his mechanical leverage back. You can see these sorts of pre- and post-postural changes online or in the offices of any ABC™ practitioner. We have many posted on our website, www.spinecentral.com. These sorts of results are typical of all ABC™ offices that use the methodology in its entirety, and they are in stark contrast to the postural improvements that many other practitioners claim to achieve.

"Posture" has become a buzz word in the chiropractic, physiotherapy and personal training worlds. Many practitioners claim to do structural correction programs, which are truly only traditional methods of manipulation or exercise followed by advice on how to hold proper posture or prescribed home stretching or tractioning exercises. If you remember from Chapter 1, this approach actually worsens one's mechanics, which is readily demonstrable by paying attention to what happens to their posture when they are instructed to completely relax (it will fold) or by observing the quality and depth of their breathing (it will be reduced) as they attempt to hold their new, muscularly controlled, "improved" posture.

This should make much more sense now that you better understand the biomechanics of compensations. Your body was already in its next-best state of balance. If you try to force it to straighten out, you are adding more compensations into the mix, which will only tighten it further and worsen your mechanics. Many of the post-treatment posture pictures of these so-called posture correction programs look forced and unnatural. You can tell that the person is holding their abdominal area in, forcibly lifting their head and chest, and pulling their shoulders down and back. The obvious point must be made that this kind of work provides temporary postural improvement at the expense of mechanical efficiency. It does not matter, however, because the results will be short-lived, and as soon at the patient stops reminding himself to hold in his abdominal area, lift his hand chest, and pull his shoulders down and back (or loses interest in continually and consciously working against gravity), he will fold back into his original compensation pattern.

There is no belief required when something is demonstrable in real time, right in front of your own eyes (or experienced through your own body, if you're the patient being corrected). When you are treated with ABC™, you will notice that it is very difficult if not outright impossible to slump forwards afterward. You will feel like you are propped upright, your shoulders down and back as though you have had a heavy load taken off of them. Your diaphragm and rib cage will be able to easily move again. One quite often experiences a lightness of mind as a calming effect floods his body, and the defence physiology lets go. Aches and pains are often significantly reduced if not eliminated after just the first treatment, and patients often report feeling lighter, and as though they "floated out of the office." What you will feel immediately after the adjustment process is a brief glimpse of the way you will consistently feel once your body has unwound through the majority of its mechanical problems.

THE UNWINDING PROCESS

So far, you have learned about all the ways your body can go wrong, and what can keep it stuck in a forwards posture. The good news is that it does not need to stay that way. There is a highly predictable and consistent journey that your body will go through when it is adjusted with the ABC™ method. We call the process unwinding, because that is, in effect, exactly what occurs overtime.

After each session, your body will immediately straighten up because we correct the out-of-place bones that the body cannot self-correct. That creates more stability. With more stability, the body can let go of the bends, twists, and rotations that it has been holding in order to compensate for the imbalances created by those out-of-place bones. Oftentimes, patients begin hearing clicks and pops throughout their body when moving around between sessions. This is their body letting go of old problems and compensation patterns and unwinding through years of built-up mechanical tension. Remember the example of the coiled-up spring? It's as though that process is being run in reverse, where one end of the spring is let go for a second, allowing it to uncoil and release stored tension. Under the surface, the new alignment and tension patterns allow the bones, ligaments, tendons, discs, muscles, and nerves of the spine to start remodeling and reworking their way into healthier, stronger, more functional configurations.

After a period of time, as you go about living your life, your body will settle into a new pattern—a deeper layer of the structural onion, so to speak. You will feel tighter and more forwards again, at which point you'll again get adjusted with the ABC™ method. You'll pop upright and go through the next phase of unwinding, getting deeper into the problem, more unwound and improved mechanically as time passes.

We know that the human body has an incredible capacity to regenerate its own tissues. Skin, for example, is replaced once per month. Liver cells are replaced every six weeks. Muscles and cartilage are replaced every three months, and bones are completely replaced every eighteen months. Your physiology is in a constant state of flux, renewing and remodeling itself on an ongoing basis in response to the demands that life places upon it.

This means that, through the corrective care process, as the structural stress patterns in your body change from abnormal to normal, tissues have the ability to regenerate back to a normal (or at least a healthier and more robust) state. One common complaint that patients present with is sciatica, which is severe back and leg pain caused by nerve pressure from a herniated disc in the lower back. Conventional medical wisdom says that it is not possible for a disc to heal completely from this sort of herniation, but this is not what we find with ABC™. The majority of patients with sciatica who go through structural correction make a full recovery over time. An ABC™ practitioner in Italy has already been able to demonstrate in two cases with pre- and post-MRIs that, after one year of care with the ABC™ methodology, a complete healing of the disc herniation had occurred. Similarly, there are case reports showing a reversal of osteoarthritis of the knee joints of patients who get unwound. These are not particularly surprising findings, given the often dramatic changes in alignment and posture that occur in every body treated with this method. More research does need to be done to be able to clearly demonstrate the amazing recuperative and regenerative powers of bodies undergoing ABC™. As more and more practitioners adopt this methodology, the scope and potential for more research should follow.

Many people say that ABC™ is "magical" because of the fast response most patients have to being corrected. While it *seems* magical given that no other form of treatment corrects *only* the out-of-place bones that the body cannot self-correct, it is not. The human body's natural response is to self-correct what it can once those things it cannot self-correct are handled. Remember, the body needs no help in being healthy; it just needs no interference to its normal function.

The length of time that it takes to correct a body's structure depends upon the complexity of the problems a person has to begin with. A child might take only a few short weeks to return to perfect posture, whereas a typical middle-aged office worker or keen athlete may take a few months to return to their best mechanical state. In general, most people will find that it provides the changes promised relatively quickly, with significant improvements noticed even after the first session.

The unwinding process itself is not always smooth sailing. Through the majority of the process, a patient will feel mechanically stable and well. During these happy times, their body is unwinding in the backwards direction where there is less stress placed upon their mechanics. As the unwinding process progresses, their spine becomes looser and "unraveled," so to speak. As this happens, the deeper-injured primary bones will be less well supported without the compensations, and will, as a result, move further forwards into their direction of injury. This temporary loss of leverage can create symptoms for a short period of time, until one's mechanics are improved enough with further treatment to bring the injured bone back into correct alignment. These symptomatic phases of care are called "forward unwinds" in ABC™ terminology, and they are a necessary and important part of the healing process, because they finally correct the injuries for which the body was initially only able to compensate. It is interesting to note that the pain of forwards unwinding will always be very similar to the pain of the injuries that the patient had historically experienced. It is quite typical for a person to come in with hip pain, for example, and say that the last time they remembered experiencing this was as a teenager after an injury. Even though a patient can be symptomatic during these forwards unwinds, by the time they experience them, they are already so much more improved mechanically that they can get along with their normal daily activities as they go through the necessary healing process. Within a couple of days to a maximum of a couple of weeks, their body will be out of its forwards unwinding phase and back into another backwards unwinding and more comfortable phase of care. Figure 7 shows the predictable healing journey of unwinding with ABC™ care.

The promise of ABC™ is that, in most cases, it will get you your life back. Things that you could easily do ten to twenty years ago that you can't do now will, usually within six months to a year, again be doable with little effort. How could this be? Well, once your body has unwound through enough of the old injuries' bends, twists, and turns that previously held it hostage, it will regain its stability and flexibility. When you reach that level of mechanical function again, you will report feeling better and healthier than you have in years, if not decades. It takes a bit longer to accomplish than to say, but it does happen and quite quickly for almost everyone.

The time it takes to correct and rehabilitate a spine with ABC™ is relatively short when you consider how long the average person has been out of balance. It does take time to regain your body's natural state, but that time is well spent since you are physically getting better with each week that passes, whereas through several other methods, you can only hope to stabilise symptomatically and attempt to stay there.

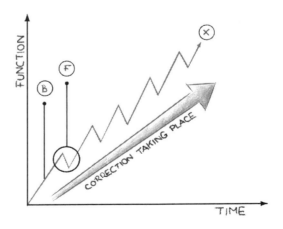

[Figure 7] The predictable and consistent progress of structural correction with more time spent unwinding. B = Backward unwind phase (feeling good). F = Forward unwind phase (feeling symptomatic). X = Fully unwound body structure with optimal alignment and function.

One of the best (and often unexpected) side effects of structural correction is the increase in body awareness that follows the improvement in posture. It's as though the brain-body connection was previously under too much stress and tension to be working properly, and now that there is less mechanical stress, there is improved communication and a heightened sense of reality. People begin to notice when they are tight or holding tension. They notice how they respond to certain foods or different shoes, beds, chairs, postures, or movements. Where you were once sleepwalking through life, you are now fully attuned to the natural feedback of your body as well as your surrounding environment. I have long considered the skill of awareness to be absolutely foundational to good health. If you can sense it, you can manage it. The remaining chapters of the book are dedicated to helping you manage and ultimately master the most important aspects of your lifestyle, which impact upon the unwinding process as well as your long-term alignment and health.

ROB'S UNWINDING STORY

Inventor, Athlete, and Entrepreneur, 37

Simply put, ABC™ changed my life. I would recommend it to anyone, whether they're suffering from serious back pain or simply wanting to feel stronger, more balanced, more fit, and future-proofed against the ageing process. After experiencing yet another episode of sciatica, I was resigning myself to limited physical recovery, unable to play sport at the level I'd like, unable to throw my nephews around the way I used to, and with the constant fear of my body failing me. It was recommended that I try ABC™, but given my past experiences with many other manual therapists, I was skeptical to say the least. The theory made sense to me, but my question was, "Would it actually do the job?"

Now that I have been through a course of care, I feel fantastic! I feel better than I did fifteen years ago. My back feels much more stable, much stronger, much more balanced. I'm not getting any pains at all, and I used to wake up every day with niggles as well as be locked up after playing sport. My tennis game is much better since my strength, flexibility, and balance have improved. I don't have to worry about playing with my nephews. Also, I recently noticed that my skiing abilities have developed to a whole new level, as better spinal alignment has led to noticeably greater balance and stability off-piste (when skiing outside of the designated ski area).

A word of warning: while some of the treatments will make you feel instantly better, some of them will bring up old injuries that the body has buried (they call it "a forwards unwind," and one of mine recreated a nervy pain in my arm that I had several years ago, which lasted a couple of weeks before vanishing forever). Work through these old injuries. Richard and his team know what they're doing, and it's a process you need to go through to get your body back to being as good as new.

CHAPTER 5

Lifestyle Choices

"We are what we repeatedly do. Excellence, then is not an act but a habit."

—*Aristotle*

A s I'm sure you're well aware by this point, the unfortunate reality is that you cannot truly fix your posture by yourself. There is no way that you can stretch, exercise, or self-manipulate in order to pull problem bones back into alignment (with one small exception that I'll share with you in a bit).

Believe me, I wish this weren't the case. Even though, as a chiropractor, I make a living helping others get their bodies back, I greatly wish that I could adjust my own body and teach others to do the same. The truth is, if you want to rebuild your body and regain lost levels of function, you are going to need to find a practitioner who uses the ABC™ method. Thankfully, there is a small army of us around the world, and the approach is growing rapidly in popularity. Chances are there is a practitioner located near you. My best advice is to go online and search your local area. If someone is an hour or two away, that's still useful, provided you have the time to invest in your health. I am constantly amazed by the fact that people will travel far and wide to visit my practice. A return journey of five hours or more is not uncommon, and people are generally extremely happy with the trade of their time for their health.

If a local practitioner isn't available, or traveling to one isn't possible for you, don't despair. You are not without options. In fact, far from it. There is a great deal that you can do to change your structural destiny. No matter how deep into the rabbit hole of complexity your issues go—in any area of health—most of the time you can track the cause of the problems back to a lifestyle choice or series of choices that were (unknowingly) made in error. There is a huge opportunity available to those who understand this and leverage it to their advantage.

Within each of these key lifestyle areas are certain small behaviours, which, if stuck with day-in and day-out, will develop into a habit. As such, they can make an out-of-proportion positive impact on your health. These habits are the small hinges that swing big doors, the twenty percent actions that bring eighty percent of the results. Let's take a look at the main areas that impact your body structure and posture long-term, and learn about the key ways to protect your alignment as you go through your days. By adopting these simple changes, you can release an enormous amount of the physical stress burden that modern life places on your body, forcing it to degenerate over time.

I am not including the following advice on how to improve the way that your stand, sit, and sleep just because I think they are good ideas or because I have seen them work for only a few people. They are included because, as with everything in the ABC™ methodology, they work consistently and predictably in the physical world. The same goes for the advice around moving your body well, except that this becomes a less predictable process since you are going to have to pay careful attention to how you move your body when you exercise. Those processes are not as easily controlled, but that does not mean that there aren't some sound principles that can guide you well. There absolutely are, and I will show you some important distinctions when it comes to exercise from the perspective of avoiding injury and strengthening your body against gravity. Put these simple principles into play, and you will support and protect your body structure far better and avoid re-injuring it as you go about your life and participate in sports.

DO YOU NEED STRAPS, TAPE, LIFTING BELTS, BACK SUPPORTS, ORTHOTICS, OR OTHER SUPPORTS?

Before we dig into the details of the habits that matter, let's address a topic that has an important connection to the advice which follows. There is a common school of thought amongst medical professions as well as sports professionals that body parts should be immobilised or restricted in order to prevent injury or prevent an existing injury from incurring further damage. Prevention of injury (or greater injury) is a valid reason to use supports, such as in the case of a fracture where a cast must be worn, or an injury whereby strapping or immobilising a body part will prevent further damage and allow continued participation by an athlete. However, if you would like to do more than just prevent further damage, it's critical to understand that inhibiting movement can hinder the body's ability to correct its own problems (or hinder the ABC™ practitioner's ability to unwind your body mechanics through its old injuries). In order to work at its peak level of performance, your body needs to be able to move freely.

The many types of support available immobilise a body part into a position that worsens the way your body moves overall rather than improves it. As is the case with a forwards-stuck bone in your spine, if you immobilise a section of your body, it will be forced to adapt with a compensation pattern, creating a chain reaction of restrictions elsewhere. This leaves you mechanically worse off.

Therefore, if you wear a restrictive support such as a wrist strap, lower back brace or knee support, or place something in your shoe to prevent your arches from collapsing, there is a tradeoff. We'll talk more about orthotics in the next chapter, but the tradeoff is between support and relief in one area and a worsening of your overall movement and structural condition. In this way, the attempted relief of one injury could set you up for many others, including poor posture and incomplete healing of injuries.

A lot goes on underneath the surface when you immobilise a joint. After just one week of not being able to move, adhesions (tissues growing together in ways that they should not) start to form, joint cartilage begins to degenerate, muscles shrink, and bones reduce in density and soften. Just ask anyone who has had their arm in a cast—it comes out of the cast six weeks later looking all sad and shriveled up, a mere shadow of its former self. It can take an additional six to twelve weeks of rehabilitation to build the tissues back up. The message is clear: movement is life, and if you stop moving part of your body, you risk losing it!

Interestingly, most people understand that when they break an arm, even though the pain is often gone (or at least significantly reduced) by the time the cast is put in place, they can't assume that the fracture has fully healed. Similarly, they do not go and play tennis immediately after taking off the cast. Doing so would be silly, and it would almost certainly cause a repeat injury. Instead, the player takes several weeks to rehabilitate his arm by doing exercises to break down adhesions and strengthen the bone, ligaments, tendons, and muscles. It will be several more weeks before he can safely get back on the court. The process of healing makes complete sense when you think about it from that perspective, yet many people tend to forget this analogy when it comes to spinal health.

A spinal joint or disc injury is often preceded by months or years of partial or complete immobilisation of a joint due to compensation tightness that progresses to leave the joint vulnerable. Please remember that once treatment has commenced and the compensation pressure is released, allowing the joints and muscles to start moving correctly, the reduction of pain that follows does not mean that healing is complete. Just as with a broken arm, there is a process that one's body must continue to go through, often for several weeks, before full strength will be regained. Remembering this can save you from falling into the re-injury trap that is so common with spine and lower back pain in particular.

There is another type of support that is becoming increasingly more commonplace, and that is the postural support strap. These straps come in various forms, from mechanical devices that connect to your phone and let you know when you are slumping to more sophisticated elasticated vests or straps that pull your shoulders down and back and literally force you to stand taller. At first glance, these devices appear to solve an important problem. But remember, there will be a tradeoff. Your breathing will likely be reduced as your body is forced into a new, major compensation pattern. Compensation always makes your body worse off mechanically, so it probably won't be long until your neck, shoulder, or back start aching. The good news is, you will probably get fed up from using these straps before they have a chance to cause any significant problems!

Generally, none of these supports are used with Advanced BioStructural Correction because the effectiveness of the adjustments and the improvements to one's biomechanics make them unnecessary—unless, of course, there is a fracture or very serious injury. No stretching and no supporting is necessary with ABC™. While it may sound too good to be true, and it certainly goes against conventional wisdom, the truth is that when you are correctly aligned, your body works so much better than much of the conventional wisdom and advice tells you. Plus, once you are correctly aligned, the ways in which you've looked after your body up until now become less relevant (even counterproductive) in most cases.

Instead, the wisest way to protect your body and allow proper healing is to avoid assuming body positions or using supports that worsen your mechanics by forcing bones out of place in directions from which the body cannot self-correct. Also, avoid restricting normal joint movement. As we've already discussed, there are many unfortunate ways this can happen through accidents and injuries, but the most common ways (by far) through which you harm your alignment and natural movement are the ways that you sit, sleep, stand, and approach your sport.

THE GENERAL RULE FOR FURNITURE AND SUPPORTS

If you want to know if your furniture is harming your body, ask yourself this simple question: Do I have difficulty getting out of it (chair, sofa, bed, car etc.) straightening up, and walking away with ease?

THE STRAIGHT TRUTH

Any time you get up off of a chair or bed and feel worse than when you sat down, that piece of furniture harmed rather than supported your alignment.

Believe it or not, the harmful consequences of common positions you assume when you engage in these everyday activities are often huge, and they create a great number of injuries to your body. The trouble is, you may not even notice them due to the condition your body has likely found itself in after years of doing things incorrectly. When your body has been stuck forwards, twisted, and locked up for many years, you are probably bound up tightly enough to endure problematic postures or tolerate modern furniture without becoming aware of any ill effects. Remember that when you get stuck forwards, adhesions form within the meningeal soft-tissue system, which in effect lock up your body. The stabilising effect of this internal tension is usually sufficient enough that you don't notice the resulting problems.

When a body is stuck forwards, it's challenging to keep it feeling comfortable. The way that modern furniture designers have worked around this problem is by producing sofas and chairs that have forward curves built into them. It seems a perfect solution to a common problem. Just look at the average sofa, chair, or recliner. The base is often soft or angled such that your bum sinks in when you sit, and the backrest is angled backwards, adding the effect that you effortlessly slump into it. This may be comfortable for a time, but it comes at a cost. If your spine is already stuck forwards, this type of chair will ensure that it stays that way (and likely develops new regions that get stuck forwards, creating a more complicated and dysfunctional body over time).

Please do not mistake this as some sort of inherent weakness in the human body. It's not that the human body is fragile; rather, it is a precision instrument, and it needs to be treated as one. The forces placed on your body from modern furniture, beds, and shoes are small but relentless. Consider how much of your day you spend sitting, standing, sleeping and moving. Those activities combined take up all twenty-four hours of the day. Get these habits wrong, and the negative impacts will add up to more than the inherent strength your body structure can resist.

If you need to use your arms to push you up out of a chair; if you feel creaky and it takes you a few moments to straighten up; if your knees, ankles, or feet feel stiff and need a few strides to loosen up; or if your neck, back, or shoulders is achy, that piece of furniture is damaging your body. It really is that simple. The same rule applies to your bed. If you wake up feeling more stiff or pained anywhere in your body than you did when you went to bed, your mattress or pillow (or often, both) is harming your body.

It doesn't matter how many thousands of dollars you have spent on your mattress or sofa, how much you love the look of it, or how well it ties the room together. If this one simple rule is broken, it is wise to listen to the message your body is sending you. Awareness of the way your body is communicating with you is such an important skill when it comes to mastering your health. Ignore it at your peril.

Interestingly, without getting your body corrected with ABC™, you run the risk of thinking the way most people think: that aches and pains are normal and they don't matter if they loosen up with some stretching and movement. Waking up with a stiff neck or getting out of a chair with a creak in your hip is often attributed to having a "pulled muscle." At this stage, you will have to take my word for it, but muscular pulling and stiffness issues associated with resting and (reasonably) normal exercise habits do not exist when true correction of your structure takes place.

Remember that when your bones are aligned correctly, your body holds itself upright with proper leverage. Muscles are no longer constantly pulling in directions they shouldn't. This means that your muscles are not under forced tension and can correctly work and relax, allowing you to sustain a good sitting, standing, or moving position for long periods of time without complaining.

By the way, the negative impact of modern furniture, mattresses, and shoes becomes extremely obvious once your body has been corrected sufficiently with ABC™ and naturally assumes its upright and relaxed alignment. If you sit on a modern sofa, you will almost immediately be able to tell that your body is being forced forwards, and it will bother you. This is partly because your spine can move so much better, and any weakness you still have will be more apparent, but it's also because you will have the benefit of contrast. You were previously in good alignment, your brain recognised what that felt like, and then you sat down and messed it up. The difference will be obvious. As I've mentioned before, this awareness is a crucial skill when working to regain optimal health and performance. Many people's awareness is dampened over time by virtue of the fact that they adapt to a new normal, one whereby their body is stiff and locked up, and they forget what it felt like to move freely. This "force of average" is something we all need to recognise and overcome in order to get the very best out of health and life. That is what we are battling, and it is going to require you to go slightly against the common grain. With that said, let's explore in greater detail at the crucial role that your feet and shoes play in your structural health.

ANNE'S UNWINDING STORY

Body and Brain Yoga Instructor, 68

Originally, I went for chronic neck pain but since that pain has gone, I have received so many other benefits. The healing journey of restoring proper alignment has been incredible. I am a body and brain yoga instructor—I had no idea how much the spine holds a key to unlocking body and brains potential. The results so far have seen improvements in my posture, sense of well-being, developing deeper sense of my body, sense of balance, breathing freely, more energy, mentally and emotionally more stable and much more able to implement healthy lifestyle changes.

Through the unwinding process they have also taught me how to better manage my diet, stress, exercise and how to look after my alignment so that I stay feeling this good. Having ABC™ treatment has significantly changed my life, I highly recommend this method, the changes you see are exceptional.

CHAPTER 6

Standing Well

"The human foot is a masterpiece of engineering and a work of art"

—*Leonardo Da Vinci*

I n this chapter, we'll cover important ground regarding the way your feet contribute to your posture and overall health. We'll look at how structural correction addresses the problem of unhealthy feet, and also the things that you can do to look after your feet through simple at-home habits. We'll explore whether or not you should be using arch supports, how to choose healthy shoes, and the one important lifestyle change that corrects and protects the health of your feet.

Many people do not realise just how important a role their feet play in their overall strength and alignment. Feet are under-appreciated, and I would argue, even abused by being imprisoned in poorly fitting shoes that do nothing to help their function and a whole lot to mess it up.

Your feet are hard workers, walking—on average—eight to ten thousand steps per day. That adds up to about 115,000 miles in a lifetime, which is impressively equivalent to no less than four times around the planet. The fact is, we were born to run, which is why the saying is so popular. Thousands of years ago, men ran huge distances in bare feet in order to catch prey. One advantage man has over animal is that he can run long distances and can also sweat to cool down. Therefore, while many animals can run faster than man, because they cannot sweat, they will tire out, and man will ultimately catch up. Anthropologists argue that this was our unique trait as predators and the reason we were able to be so successful as a species, especially early on. Many aspects of our mechanical design are uniquely suited to running and walking. We are born masters of these domains, and we will do it naturally very well if our body mechanics are working correctly.

Each time your foot strikes the ground, the impact force that is placed back up through your feet, knees, hips, and spine can be many times greater than your body weight. Consider that your feet are the faithful warriors of your everyday existence, bearing forces totaling hundreds of tons on any given day as you move around your world. The only way that they can do this without falling apart is with thanks to some impressive natural engineering.

Surely you agree that it's impossible to consider any part of the human body and not be impressed by the perfection of its design and the way it so perfectly aids its function, but this is especially true when it comes to the foot. The result of seven million years of evolutionary progress, the foot is an amazing example of natural engineering at its finest. They are each packed with an intricate network of 26 bones, 33 joints, 3 arches, 107 ligaments, and 19 muscles and tendons that come together to form a highly sensitive, flexible, robust, and adaptable machine.

Your feet are charged with the awesome task of providing support to your skeleton and absorbing and distributing the shock of your movements. They must also relay critical information to your brain, letting it know how you are moving, what you are standing on, and how to move next. This complicated and dynamic interplay between support, movement, and brain signaling is what allows you to stand, walk, run, and perform all manner of complex tasks gracefully, almost regardless of terrain.

Since structure determines function, your foot can only do its job well when it's properly aligned. Just as weak foundations caused the Tower of Pisa to lean, weak feet can upset the balance of your whole body, becoming a significant and continual source of stress that the rest of your body has to adapt to. This means that regaining full function of your feet is a critical piece of the health puzzle, and if you look after them well, they will have no problem supporting you for a lifetime.

HOW GOOD IS YOUR SENSE OF BALANCE?

To get an idea of how important brain-to-joint communication is to structural health, try this experiment. Put on your running shoes, close your eyes, and stand on one leg. Count the number of seconds for which you can remain steady before you start to wobble and fall. Then, take off your shoes and socks and repeat the experiment. What do you notice? If you are like most people, you'll notice that you are significantly more stable when barefoot. Notice as you do the test just how dynamic your foot is in the process of simply standing still. It will efficiently and precisely change the position of the foot arches, toes, and heel bone with subtle muscle contractions that maintain your centre of gravity. This is how your feet—literally the foundations of your body—work to keep you in balance.

FOOT STRESS

You may not have heard this term before, but foot stress is a very real form of physical stress that, over time, has negative effects on whole body health. Foot stress is pandemic throughout the developed world because, from a young age, we are socially conditioned to imprison our feet in tightly fitting, inflexible shoes.

This can be very unhealthy for the foot and the structure as a whole, resulting in a gradually stiffened and misaligned foot. Conditions like bunions, hammer toes, claw toes, and hyper-pronation are likely to be created by poor footwear choices that, over time, contort and distort the foot mechanics.

It's interesting to think that our hunter-gatherer ancestors thrived for millions of years without any form of elaborate or sophisticated footwear. In fact, if our genes expect anything at all from us, it is that we should be barefoot. It makes sense that seven million years of standing on two legs has installed some design features that should allow the foot to sense the ground on which it stands, and be strong and flexible enough to walk, hike, sprint, and even run long distances barefoot. The human foot is designed to be free, to be moved, to be challenged with regular physical activity, and to be in contact with the ground as often as possible. These days, however, we are socially conditioned to wear something on our feet at all times, essentially shielding them from the environment beneath. By blocking free foot movement and numbing feedback from the ground, you also impede the sensing activity of nerves in the foot. This ultimately results in distorted and reduced communication between the body and brain, leaving people less able to quickly adapt to the demands of movement and more prone to injury.

When you deeply study the human body, one of the fascinating things that stands out is how completely interconnected it is. All of your systems, subsystems, and various anatomical parts are intimately interconnected and reliant upon each other for their continued proper functioning as well as continued proper functioning of the body as a whole. Posture, for one, is partially automatically controlled by the alignment and leverage of your foot bones as well as the proprioceptive feedback to your brain from the nerves in your feet. If the foot becomes de-conditioned, so does posture, which will cause you to begin to stoop and slump forwards. Healthy knee, hip, pelvis, and lower back alignment is also highly interdependent. The foot muscles, for example, get information on how to work from the nerves of your lower back, so misalignments in the base of your spine can cause numerous foot weaknesses and problems over time. As an example, the main medial arch of the foot is supported and maintained by the action of the posterior tibialis muscles, which are supplied from nerves that exit the base of your spine. Through this direct anatomical connection, a lower-back problem can cause a foot to hyper-pronate.

Coordinated movements of your lower back and lower limb muscles when you stand, walk, and run are, in turn, highly dependent upon proprioceptive feedback from the foot and ankle nerve cells. What this means is that you rarely just get a lower back problem or a foot problem—in fact, you rarely get *any* problem in isolation. Everything is intricately interconnected. We are an ecosystem of cells, and each part of us has a vital and equally important role to play in the health of the whole. No part can be neglected.

DO YOU NEED ORTHOTICS?

One of the common theories as to why feet "go wrong" is that they pronate, or roll inwards. Therefore, one of the questions that I'm frequently asked is, "Should I be wearing orthotics?" In case you don't know what orthotics are, they are toughened arch supports that you wear inside your shoes to stop your feet from rolling inwards. Sometimes they're custom made for your feet, and sometimes they are purchased off the shelf as generic designs. Often, a degree of arch support is built into running shoes, and although these are not technically an orthotic, they work in the same way.

The conversation around whether or not to wear them is

surprisingly complex, but it ultimately comes down to how you want your body to get better, functionally or symptomatically. Before we dive deeper into the topic, I want to be clear that there is no doubt that orthotics can be of significant help to people with over-pronated feet. If the orthotics are correctly fitted, they can provide relief for back, hip, knee, and foot complaints. The question of whether or not this is good or bad comes down to what you are trying to achieve. By wearing an orthotic, you may take pressure out of a painful area, but you'll also shift pressure into another area. This may or may not lead to other symptoms, but it will always worsen your mechanics. Another issue is that, if orthotics *do* help you, you'll have a crutch that you'll have to continue using for the rest of your life, and the more you wear them, the more you'll need them because your foot gets weaker when it's supported.

Because your feet are such an important part of your overall structure, they need to be cared for and conditioned alongside the rest of the of your body. Your feet, as important as they are, do not work in isolation from the rest of your bones. Remember that your entire skeleton is a single synchronised functioning unit, and a change in one area will immediately affect all other areas. So your back will affect your feet, and your feet will affect your back, and so on.

Remember meninges? They're the strong, elastic, flexible tissues that cover your brain and spinal cord, and when postures get stuck forwards, they can get stretched and scarred against the inside of the spinal column, effectively anchoring your body into poor alignment. This internal tension can protect against further damage, but at the same time it creates a tensioning of the entire body, changing the way that you work mechanically from head to toe. The neurosurgeon, Dr. Yamada (who I introduced to you in Chapter 3), discovered this unexpectedly when foot deformities were corrected as a side effect in sixty-one percent of patients who had undergone surgical untethering of their spinal cord—a lower-back surgery that involves cutting the meninges in order to slacken the adverse tension they're placing on the spinal cord. This means that any discussion of foot alignment must take into account the meninges alongside the other bones of your legs, pelvis, and spine.

Even in this day and age, there is still great debate as to what exactly an orthotic should look like and how it should work. The science is by no means clear cut for one simple reason: most of the studies that have been done focus purely on the foot with the intent to tackle the sole issue (pun intended) of stabilising the rolling in (or pronation), which is considered to be the problem that needs solving. However, no consideration is given to how the rest of the body factors into the situation.

The conversation is further complicated by the many opinions and theories as to what a "normal" foot alignment should be. Then there is also the issue of how one should cast the orthotic, which begs questions regarding whether the recipient should be seated and not weight-bearing or standing *and* weight-bearing as well as whether they should be cast one at a time or together. These factors are all questioned in the research alongside multiple theories on the size, shape, flexibility, and material of the orthotic and what sort of "ideal" alignment an orthotic should place the foot into. All of these variables confirm that even with the extensive research available, there are no firm conclusions, and people's results after wearing orthotics are often inconsistent as well.

Much of the confusion is minimised when you consider the fact that pronation is a natural part of healthy foot movement. The three arches of your foot stretch and elongate as you put weight on it, dissipating the shock and giving a spring-like effect that propels you forwards. It's clever, natural engineering that allows you to control your weight and the reactive forces from the ground. You *need* your arches to change shape as you move; this is part of their ideal design.

There is, however, a difference between pronation and over-pronation. Over-pronation is a real issue, and it causes significant problems for some people. There are cases, especially in older individuals, where the integrity of the arch has been lost to a significant enough degree that mechanical stability is insufficient and unable to be fully regained. Whilst these more severe cases can be improved with structural correction, the process will take longer. Rehabilitation will be required to find stability, and results may never be complete. So, if you have significantly pronated feet, an orthotic may help to stabilise your pain and allow you to live your life more fully. It is certainly easier and quicker than trying to rehabilitate your feet back to full health, although you will almost certainly be able to regain some of the lost function if you follow the advice given in this chapter.

Since your whole body works together, if ABC™ can correct your posture, it stands to reason that it can help your feet as well. It is actually often not possible to correct posture without correcting mechanical foot problems. The same mechanical principles at work in the spine are true of the feet and legs. Foot bones can also go out of alignment in directions from which they cannot be retrieved because there are no muscles to do that job. They therefore require mechanical force in the form of an adjustment to get back into alignment. Foot bones can also misalign as part of a compensation pattern for problems elsewhere in the body, just as can forwards-stuck bones in the lower back. This explains the common scenario whereby people have back pain while sitting down but feel much better when standing up. Their legs and feet twist up to compensate for the mechanical stress in the lower back, making it feel better.

Here is another experiment that you can do on yourself and your family members. Stand up and march in place for a few seconds. Then stop and look down at your feet. You will likely see one foot turned further outwards than the other. You will notice the same thing if you lie on your back and lift your head to look down at your feet; the same foot will be turned out further. This is the compensation twist that your body builds in to protect itself mechanically. If you have good body awareness, you will notice that this is the same side on which your hip feels tighter, since it is predominantly the hip flexor muscle (known as the iliopsoas) that tightens up in this scenario.

The interconnectedness of the entire human frame is rarely considered by those who prescribe orthotics (that can cost upwards of £600 for custom-moulded pairs) or in the currently available research studies. This makes it is entirely possible that you could stand on an orthotic and actually *worsen* your overall mechanics by taking out or changing a compensation pattern that was helping to stabilise you. People often wear orthotics and get relief of their foot pain only to develop hip, knee, or back pain a week or so later. Many practitioners chalk this up to the body going through an "adaptation phase", but there is more going on than that. When your body works well mechanically, you do not notice it; it quietly gets on with its job.

Orthotics can also cause problems for people going through true structural correction. I have had many patients over the years who have made good progress initially, only to eventually plateau and fail to progress further. This scenario is always surprising when practicing with ABC™ because the body should continue to change over time as mechanical problems are corrected. In the cases where they don't, it's either because something incorrect is being done clinically (perhaps the practitioner is inexperienced or missing a key adjustment) or the patient is doing something to recreate the same problems and impede progress. More often than not, it's the latter. A common issue I find is that patients are wearing orthotics that were prescribed by a previous practitioner, and they neglect to mention it. When the orthotics are removed and their feet are allowed to move naturally, their bodies continue to unwind and they return to making excellent progress with their structural correction. These same patients are also surprised to discover that they now function just fine *without* their orthotics, now that their body is doing so much better mechanically.

WHAT WE KNOW TO BE TRUE ABOUT SUPPORTING YOUR FEET

Dr. Jutkowitz carried out research on the use of foot orthotics and their impact upon whole body alignment. He used pre and post full-spine X-ray analysis to mathematically measure the structural changes that occur when orthotics are worn. Unfortunately, this research has yet to published, but I will talk about it to both illustrate the point and show you that my recommendations are far from baseless. These points are easy to verify on patients in real time, which I have done many times over. You can test these points on yourself as well.

The first notable takeaway from Dr. Jutkowitz's research was that any support under the ball of the foot worsens your spinal mechanics. Therefore, any support that raises the base of your toes will make your overall alignment worse. Most orthotics, which aim to support all three of the foot arches, will do this, as will the insoles in many trainers. The same effect can also occur if the heel area of the shoe sinks in, causing the heel bone to tilt backwards and the toes to become relatively higher than the heel. This effect is known as a "negative heel," and it is very common in modern shoes due to their cushioned sole, especially once they are worn in.

Years ago, before I understood this concept, I bought a pair of running shoes that had a raised support under the base of the toes, also known as the transverse arch of the foot. They were marketed as better for running by helping to propel you forwards and cushion the impact. They ended up a complete disaster for me, causing all kinds of knee and hip pain after just a few weeks of use. This led me on a long path of trying to figure out why I was getting injured. It took ages and a lot of money and frustration to determine that nearly all high-tech modern running shoes can cause problems of one sort or another. It wasn't until I started using minimalist shoes without any kind of arch support that I was able to overcome my running injury woes. One of the key lessons I've learned is that despite the multi-million-dollar marketing messages of shoe companies, there is nothing that you can put in a shoe that will improve upon the function of the human foot. A classic study published in *British Journal of Sports Medicine* concluded that "expensive athletic shoes are deceptively advertised to safeguard well through cushioning impact, yet account for 123% greater injury than the cheapest ones."[31]

Here is how you can test out the theory yourself. Take a breath in and notice its depth and quality as well as the balance point of your neck and shoulders. Then, stand up and place a thin book lengthwise under the ball (front) of each foot and take in a breath. You will likely notice that your breath is more restricted with less depth and freedom of movement, and your neck and head are thrown forwards slightly to compensate. If you don't notice it, try this exercise again with a thicker book. Anything that raises the base of the toes relative to the heel will harm your posture.

The second key finding of his research was that no matter a person's mechanical condition, good or bad, heels always improve biomechanics.

This is another important discovery, and it won't be terribly surprising to women who claim that wearing heels actually helps their back pain. The reason it works is that raising the heel height tips the top of the pelvis forwards, increasing the angle between it and the lower back bones. This improves your body's ability to lever itself upright against gravity.

The positive benefit is seen with a heel height primarily between zero (flat) and one and a half inches. How much further a person can go above that range before starting to overcompensate and have postural problems (usually the upper chest is thrown forwards) depends upon a particular body's unique alignment pattern.

The use of heels is a solution to consider since it is cheap and easy to purchase thin heel lifts and place them at the back of your shoes. Practically speaking, most people require a heel in the range of 2 - 6mm, making it a fairly precise thing to tinker with. The best way to get this right is to have your local ABC™ practitioner take a look at shoes and make the corrections while observing the impact made on your body's balance and posture (See Figure 8).

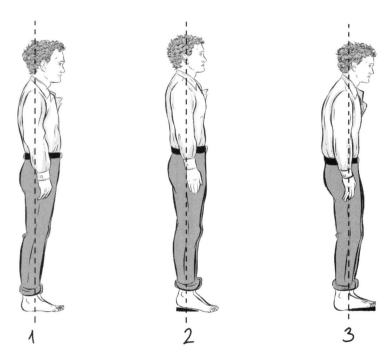

[Figure 8:1] Standing with no heel lift and a body structure that has some misalignment. Note the slight forwards lean.

[Figure 8:2] Standing with a heel lift of less that 1.5 inches. Note the ideal alignment with the body centered on the plumb line.

[Figure 8:3] Standing with a lift under the front of the foot (which is what happens when your heels sink down into the sole of a shoe). Note the shift of the pelvis slightly backwards while the upper back is pushed forwards.

HOW TO CHOOSE HEALTHY SHOES

We've made some big strides forwards so far in understanding feet (see what I did there?), beginning with the premise that your feet are designed to pronate, and they work with the rest of your body, not independent from it. If you want your body to get better over time, you must allow your feet to move freely, without restriction or hindrance.

THE STRAIGHT TRUTH

There is nothing you can put into a shoe that will improve the way your foot works.

It's already an engineering miracle in and of itself, and as such, all it needs is to be allowed to work the way nature intended. To achieve this, you must choose shoes that are designed to accommodate the healthy function of the foot rather than restrict it. The vast majority of modern footwear does not allow your foot to feel the ground or bend and move freely. Over time, this causes mechanical restrictions and weaknesses that can leave you vulnerable to injuries through a loss of both structural strength and overall kinesthetic sense from your feet to your brain. One of the best habit changes you can make is to start wearing foot friendly shoes.

Before we dive into the basics of a healthy shoe, let's have a look at a few key terms that are important to understand when it comes to choosing good footwear.

Stack height is the distance between the point at which the shoe touches the floor and that at which your foot touches the shoe. Generally, the greater the stack height, the more cushioning there will be in the shoe.

That leads us to the next term, **drop height**, which is the difference in height from the back of the shoe to the front. For example, if the rear stack height were 3cm and the front stack height were 1cm, the drop height would be 2cm.

Next is the **toe-box**, which is the amount of room in the front of the shoe allowing your forefoot to move. Many modern shoe designs have a narrow toe box, causing the toes to squash together like a pencil point rather than be allowed to fan out and move. If you look at pictures of healthy feet, you will see that the front of the foot is wide and the toes fan out so as not to touch each other. On the other hand, after years of wearing tight shoes, a foot can become tight and misaligned, and the forefoot will appear narrowed with the toes squished together.

The next measurement, the most common one, is **shoe size**. Many people buy shoes that are the wrong size for their feet. If your shoe is too small, your big toe will jam up against the end of the shoe, and that can cause a lot of problems. If your toenails feel or look bruised after long runs or walks, there is a good chance that your shoes are too small. If you buy shoes that are too big, your foot will slide and you will get muscular compensation problems in your calf and foot muscles. The moral of the story is, get the basics right, and have your feet measured.

Interestingly, I have had many patients over the years, including myself, claim that their feet have grown by up to one-and-a-half sizes after being treated with ABC™ for a few months alongside changing to foot- friendly shoes. When you fix the bones that the body cannot self-correct and allow the joints to move freely, the foot will "unwind" back into its ideal alignment, allowing the forefoot to open up and the toes to spread and stretch out. Most people's feet are a far cry from what they should be. Years of wearing the wrong shoes will cause the toes to squash together and the foot to narrow and tighten. When you address these key issues, you can expect some significant changes to the way your feet look and function over time.

The next concept to understand is the **flexibility** of the shoe, how much it twists and bends in ways that are natural to a human foot. The more flexible it is, the better. This advice is contrary to conventional wisdom, which says that you must support the foot in order to stop it from bending too much in order to avoid injuries such as twisted ankles. Interestingly, the science doesn't support this. In fact, the evidence suggests that the more supportive a shoe is, the greater the likelihood that you will experience injury. Your foot needs to move well in order to provide proprioceptive feedback to your brain so that you can control your limbs properly, adapt to changes in terrain, and avoid injuries. Wearing stiff and/or over-cushioned shoes not only reduces this kinesthetic sense but also leads to a gradual weakening of your feet. Once again, it's a case of move it or lose it. A healthy everyday shoe should be able to bend easily in all directions and at all points, including twisting. Obviously, if you are going to be hiking over difficult, rugged terrain, your needs may be different in that specific instance.

FOOT SENSE

We are all familiar with the senses of smell, taste, and sight. Foot sense is not as well known a sense, but it is equally important. Every time your foot hits the floor, your brain needs to know exactly how to adapt your body to absorb the forces and react to any changes in the terrain. If you step on a sharp stone, the body reacts by immediately contracting certain muscles that lift your foot off the ground and away from the danger. Known as the withdrawal reflex, this automatic safety system has likely saved you from injuring yourself many times in your life. This is an example of foot sense in action; it allows you to maintain your balance and dignity and avoid unfortunate trips, injuries, or sprains.

Your brain can only perform this important job when the foot structure is well-aligned, and your choice of footwear allows your foot to move and correctly sense the ground. This simple physiological fact is often overlooked, and the wrong choice of footwear can significantly impede the function of your feet, causing long-term, harmful effects to your posture and overall robustness. The message is simple: if you want to prevent injuries and unlock levels of performance and robustness that have eluded you so far, pay attention to your feet and the way you treat them on a day-to-day basis.

Foot sense is enabled by the millions of highly specialised nerve endings embedded in the tissues of your feet, which are among the most nerve-enriched areas of the whole body. These nerves are located within the muscles, skin, ligaments, and joints where they detect tension, movement, force, pressure, and temperature changes in the foot. The scientific term for this kind of nerve communication is proprioception, which comes from the Latin word *proprius,* meaning "one's own," and the English word perception. It is often referred to as the sixth-sense because it is an awareness of the relative position of your body parts as well as the effort you are using while moving. Without proprioception, you wouldn't be able to move because your brain would have no idea how to instruct the movements since it wouldn't know where your body parts were to begin with!

There are a few unfortunate people around the world who have contracted a rare, degenerative condition of the nervous system whereby they lose their proprioceptive sense completely and are effectively left paralysed, even though the motor nerve supply to their muscles is left unaffected. Without an awareness of the starting position of a joint, the brain is rendered unable to move without extreme concentration. Imagine if simply gesturing whilst you spoke became as complicated and energy intensive as juggling? That is what it is like for people who cannot feel their joint movements. They have to learn to control themselves as they would control a TV by remote control; one wayward move can send them crashing to the floor.

Proprioception is crucial to everything you do that involves movement. When your proprioceptive nerves fire, information is sent to the brain, which is used to work out the relative positions of neighbouring body parts. Instructions can then be sent to your muscles to adapt your movement and posture accordingly. Amazingly, this goes on continuously and automatically without you ever having to think about it.

With every step you take, the foot automatically senses information about the ground relative to your posture. Your brain then uses this data to make changes to body. The pebble in your shoe may cause you to adjust your foot angle, or a blister might cause you limp in order to alleviate the pain. As your foot continues to assess information about pressure, force, tension, and movement, it sends this information along nerves, through the spinal cord, and up to the brain. Your brain uses this information to allow your entire body to respond to this foot sense. This body-wide sense is your kinesthetic sense. It is because of kinesthetic sense that you don't need to look down at your feet to know where they are; your brain automatically senses their location.

HOW TO OPTIMISE YOUR FOOT SENSE AND STRENGTH

The key to optimising your foot sense is either to go barefoot or to wear shoes that are as close to barefoot as possible. Unless you can feel the ground, and unless your foot can move freely, there will be a dampened ability to sense, which causes a reduced ability to adapt and control your body.

The final point to understand about shoes is with regard to all of the "**technology**" that gets put inside of them. Oftentimes, that technology comes by way of one of two guises, the first of which is **cushioning**, or the amount that your foot "squashes" into the shoe. There's all manner of technology, from air cells to pumps and gel packs, that are built into shoes, mostly because they make them more comfortable. Just as a soft mattress is required for a tightly twisted spine to get comfortable, a tightly twisted foot is more comfortable on a soft surface. When your body is corrected with ABC™ and the twist comes out, it needs adequate support in order to stay well-aligned. Soft trainers will work against this development and cause foot problems to come back.

The other reason that trainers are cushioned stems from the faulty idea that, despite a few million years of evolution, the foot needs extra help to avoid the impact of walking and exercising. Therefore, extra cushioning and support are provided. I realise that it's somewhat ridiculous to try to achieve both, but that's what happens. So there is a whole spectrum of cushioning added to shoes, none of which has ever been shown to reduce injuries in athletes. In fact, the research shows the opposite. The more high-tech and cushioned a trainer is, the greater the likelihood of injury. Interestingly, a 2018 study found that maximally cushioned running shoes actually *increased* rather than lessened the impact forces in the lower limbs[32], probably because they encourage a running style that relies on the trainer rather than the runner's own efficient movement. Studies also showed that when a less-cushioned trainer is used, fewer injuries are experienced.[33] Again, this is likely because it encourages the athlete to run on the mid-forefoot rather than strike heavily through the heel. That is one of the main problems of wearing cushioned shoes: they encourage you to heel strike, which is not the way the foot is designed to work.

You can once again test this out for yourself by putting on a pair of cushioned trainers and going for a run. Notice how you instinctively stride out and land on your heel bone. Then, take your shoes off completely (you might want to do this in the park or garden where the ground is slightly softer), and go for a short run. Notice how your body works completely differently, and that you naturally land on the forefoot or mid-foot in a light, controlled way. Once again, not only your foot but also your full body mechanics work naturally and instantly better when your foot can freely move and sense the ground beneath. Also, once you have worn in these sorts of shoes, there is often a "negative heel" created in the base of the shoe where your heel bone sinks in. This causes the foot to tilt the wrong way, and it will further harm your biomechanics and posture as previously explained.

Poor posture and poor biomechanics will also encourage you to heel strike when you run. I mentioned earlier my fascination with watching the movement and posture of children. Up until the age of four or five, they move with perfect form. They run like Olympic sprinters, mechanically sound and technically perfect, landing on the front of their feet—regardless of whether they are running fast or slow. Yet, somewhere between the ages of five and six, many start to adopt a different technique, slamming their heels into the ground when running. You have to wonder what happened during this time. Why would a child who instinctively knew how to run well go through such a dramatic shift in movement mechanics? The answer is explained through the changes that their bony structure goes through during this first year of school, when they first begin their sitting career. Recently, an Australian chiropractor by the name of Dr. James Carter made headlines when he published X-ray studies of children as young as seven already showing reverse spinal curves as a result of sitting and using their smartphones too often. These images are still available online if you're interested in seeing them.

The second type of technology added to shoes is **arch supports**. There are various sizes and types, and they are placed at different locations through the three arches of the foot. The most common arch support is the medial arch support, or inner arch support, in the middle part of the foot. Remember, there is nothing that can be put under the foot to improve the way it inherently works. In fact, from a pure engineering point of view, the worst place to support an arch is the middle. Think of an old-fashioned arched stone bridge, for example. If you put upward pressure on the keystone section of an arch (which represents the mid-foot in this analogy), all you actually do is weaken the natural strength of that arch, leaving it vulnerable to collapse. This is why it makes very little sense to put a support under the mid-foot and suggest that it's improving the foot's function.

CHOOSING A HEALTHY SHOE (SUMMARY)

If you can get all of the following boxes checked off, you will be giving your feet the best possible chance of regaining strength and flexibility over time.

1. The best shoes have thin (low) stack height and no drop from back to front. It is best to avoid thickly cushioned shoes. Many shoes have arch supports built into the inner sole. You can usually pull these out. If they are not removable, you will need to buy new shoes. The shoe may feel too big when the inner sole is removed, and if that happens, simply purchase a flat inner sole to replace it.

2. The height of the heel does not matter too much. A small heel of up to 1.5 inches can be beneficial for your overall posture. Try to avoid heels greater than 1.5 inches high, as they can throw off your

entire postural balance by tipping your pelvis excessively forwards. You will have to pay attention to what your body is doing when you wear high heels. If you feel that your upper back and neck are thrown forwards, the heel is too high.

3. A more common problem with many modern shoes is that they have a "negative heel," meaning that the very back of the heel dips downwards causing the heel bone (calcaneus) to sink and your posture to fail forwards. An ABC™ practitioner will be able to check your shoes and let you know if this problem is occurring, but you can usually tell by running your fingers along the inner sole and noticing if it dips down at the back. A negative heel is also commonly found in shoes that have been worn down over time through overuse.

4. Avoid shoes such as "cross trainers," which often have permanent arches already moulded into the shoe. Wearing these shoes will stop your body from unlocking and unwinding by blocking normal foot mechanics. Some popular brands of moulded, cork-soled sandals can cause problems, as can shoes with a curved sole intended to make one's body constantly rock in order to engage muscles.

5. Make sure that your shoes are wide enough in the toe box, and that the toe of the shoe is not squeezing your toes together. Your forefoot needs room to move so that your arches and toes can spread out as you bear weight.

6. Make sure that your shoes are long enough to avoid squashing your big toe against the end of the shoe. Not only can this harm the big toe joint, it can also have a significantly negative effect on the way that your whole body moves. Ensure that there is at least 1 cm of room between the end of the big toe and the end of the shoe.

7. If you are undergoing treatment with ABC™ technique and you know your breakdown side (everybody has a breakdown side, either left or right, that their body tends to fall towards under mechanical stress), you can help support that breakdown side by placing a small lift under the arch of that foot. For example, if your breakdown side is the left, you would only support the left arch. Do this by taping together two plasters lengthwise, one on top of the other, and placing them on your inner sole so that the pads are under the highest part of your arch. Some people only require one plaster; some require three. Start with two, and test them out by walking while paying attention to your posture. Make adjustments if necessary. The size seems quite small, especially compared to modern orthotics, but it is enough to support you mechanically with the understanding that your arches are supposed to flatten out a bit as you move. You can test out the theory by placing the support on the wrong foot and noticing the differences. If you are not undergoing structural correction and do not know your breakdown side, you can still try the experiment to see if you notice a benefit to supporting one foot over the other. If you can, this approach should help you. If you can't, don't worry. It is a finer correction, and you should manage well without it.

BAREFOOT THERAPY

After years of imprisonment in unhelpful shoes, it is likely that your feet have become weakened and will hugely benefit from rehabilitation and ongoing maintenance. Human beings have been evolving for millions of years, yet it is only in the last 40,000 of those years that we have been wearing shoes. And only in the last thirty of those years have we been experimenting with cushioning and support technology. The poor condition of many people's feet is yet another reflection of how our modern environments no longer match our biology. Any time we are out of alignment with our innate genetic blueprint, there is a price to pay, and that price is the loss of functional health.

The best way to recondition your feet is through barefoot therapy, which is a process of gradually reintroducing the types of movement and conditions that your feet evolved to work best in. When it comes to rebuilding your feet, the key is not to do too much too soon. Just as it takes many months to safely prepare for a marathon, it can take many months to strengthen your feet to the point where they can handle a barefoot run, hike, or other sport. There is no doubt that you will have many weakened and shrunken tissues that need to be rebuilt. Don't risk failure and injury by rushing the process. You don't want to overwhelm the tissues of your feet by doing too much too soon. Give your muscles and tendons a chance to adapt and recover, and as the weeks and months roll by, your feet will gradually strengthen and start to provide you with the enormous benefits that come from optimal kinesthetic sense and foot strength. As time goes on, you will start to notice that you feel rooted to the floor with a degree of strength, stability, and agility that was previously not there. If you get ABC™ alongside introducing barefoot therapy your results will come faster and be amplified greatly.

STEPS TO RESTORING FOOT STRENGTH AND FLEXIBILITY

1. Take off your shoes and socks daily. Do this for at least ten minutes and walk around the house. Break the habit of putting socks, slippers, and shoes on in the morning. Take your shoes off first thing when you get home. Try to spend as much time as you can standing, walking, and otherwise being barefoot in your home, office, and other indoor locations. It is best to wear no socks at all, but wearing a thin pair will still produce good results. This is the first step to rehabilitating your feet. Don't underestimate how effective this can be at starting to rehabilitate foot problems if you have had your feet imprisoned in supportive and/or restrictive shoes for a lifetime. Do this for a couple of weeks, spending as much time barefoot as you can each day before progressing to the next step.

2. Walk outside barefoot. Take the plunge. Head outside and walk around on different surfaces. The additional challenge and stimulation that this provides to the nerves and muscles of the foot are important to the foot's rehabilitation. Initially, you may wish to stick to smoother surfaces such as the road or your driveway, but don't shy away from gravel or roughened concrete. Harsher surfaces really help speed up the learning process in terms of how you distribute your weight across the sole of your foot. Bending your knees a bit can help make it more comfortable. Aim for ten minutes of outside barefoot walking (regardless of the time of year) as well as continuing with Step One. After about a week, you will be ready to move on. The rougher the surface, the better. You will appreciate this later on, once you start to do more advanced workouts since your natural technique will be so much better. Don't worry if your foot appears to be hypersensitive at the beginning. Soon the skin will toughen up, and the sensitivity level will dial down. Eventually, you will be able to walk across gravel without even thinking about it.

3. Start wearing minimal shoes most of the time. During the times when you cannot be truly barefoot, such as when you're at work, running, shopping, or socialising, wear minimal shoes that provide conditions close to being barefoot. Build the length of time you spend in minimal shoes up to an hour or more daily. When you can spend a full hour in minimal shoes (or even barefoot), your foot is probably strong enough to begin doing sports and more vigorous exercises barefoot or with minimal footwear. The good news is that, today, the minimal shoe market is really taking off. There is a definite trend toward searching out more natural ways of training, and as a result, there are some really good options available that will allow you to live the barefoot lifestyle most of the time.

At the time of writing, Vivobarefoot is a fantastic company that supplies a whole range of minimalist footwear for all aspects of daily life, from work to street wear to sportswear. Vibram is another company whose shoes (including the infamous FiveFingers design shoe) provide perhaps the closest possible experience to being barefoot whilst wearing shoes. Xero Shoes is another brand who provide both casual and sporty options.

The beauty of these minimal shoes is that they fulfill most, if not all, of the criteria of a healthy shoe (you could easily insert a heel lift into them if you wanted or needed to). With a simple, thin film of rubber that covers the sole of your foot, protecting it from anything sharp or unsavoury that you may walk or run over, you are able to move freely but also feel what is beneath your feet with a much higher degree of sensitivity than you can while wearing most modern shoes. They are very light as well, so you hardly notice that you are wearing them.

There are many other shoe companies such as Skora, Merrell, New Balance, Saucony, Nike, and Adidas, to name but a few that have started to produce minimal shoes. The best approach is to go to a specialist running store and try a few different varieties. It doesn't hurt to have more than one pair. So experiment and find what works well for you and your feet, but avoid the trap of trying to find a pair that feels really "comfortable" to begin with, because that usually means that they are too cushioned. A foot-friendly shoe will just get on with its job without you noticing it much one way or another.

When I first started transitioning to barefoot training, I found that I could only spend a certain amount of time in minimalist shoes before my foot and calf muscles started to ache. A useful approach is to always have options available. Take your minimal trainers on your hike and wear them for thirty minutes at a time on sections where the surface is gentle. If you end up on terrain that is rougher and rockier, simply switch back to your old shoes for some added protection. Over time, your feet will strengthen, and you will be able to wear minimalist shoes most of the time. These days, I run, play tennis, hike, do all of my workouts, and spend my entire working day in minimalist shoes. When your foot becomes accustomed to "feeling" the floor, you will find this sort of sensation quite addictive. In fact, if I wear fancy leather dress shoes or conventional trainers these days, I experience what can only be described as foot stress, which not only negatively affects my gait, posture, and feet but also my state mind. I find it mildly irritating and distracting to have my foot squeezed into an overly tight or cushioned shoe. Most ABC™ clients who follow this advice report the same surprising discovery. Foot sense and proprioception can be considered essential nutrients, and once you have the contrast in your mind, it will be difficult to tolerate going backwards.

This strange phenomenon of wellness living is not exclusively reserved for minimal trainers. It seems to occur anytime you remove a significant stressor for a period of time and then reintroduce it. Alcohol is a good example. Once you remove it for a few weeks, the next drink you consume will have an out-of-proportion impact on how you feel. The same occurs with positive dietary changes, periods of regular exercise, or frequent meditation. It is as though your body gets addicted to functioning well and amplifies the regression warning signs to help you keep it that way.

4. Self-care for your tired feet. Anyone can start to add in the first steps of barefoot therapy. As you get more and more active with barefoot living, you may find that your feet start to get tired and achy. Gentle foot massages can go a long way when it comes to helping speed your progress along at this point. Pay a professional or do it yourself at home by rolling the sole of your foot lightly over a golf ball. Just explore your foot. It may be painful at first, but that just means it's working. Finding the sore pressure points and hold them until you feel a release. Try flexing, extending, and moving your toes around as you roll over the tight spots. Lastly, try to put your foot through every possible range and type of motion that it might experience in the real world. Engaging in a few minutes of this each night can be very beneficial for your feet.

Remember that getting true structural correction with ABC™ will usually immediately remove any sensation of muscular tightness or achiness in your feet and calves. If you can't get adjusted with this method, and if you are taking barefoot therapy seriously, a certain degree of self-care can be helpful, but it is not required. If you do choose to massage your own feet, be gentle. The compensation tightness in your feet is also doing a job of stabilising your whole structure, so try to keep self-massage to a minimum and avoid deep tissue style therapies. A period of rest is often enough to fully recover from the effects of barefoot therapy.

5. Foot-strengthening exercises. You should be able to easily stand on one leg for thirty to sixty seconds with your eyes open. If you can manage only ten seconds or less before you fall, it is likely that you have a foot imbalance that could be significantly improved with practice. By balancing on each foot, you can gradually improve the communication between the brain and the feet. Over time, this will lead to better overall balance throughout the whole body.

An easy way to add this practice into your lifestyle is, when you get out of the shower, hold one foot up to dry it whilst you balance on the other. Hold for as long as you can, and then repeat on the other side. You can do something similar when you put on your shoes or are waiting for the kettle to boil, or when working at a stand-up desk (my personal favourite). This exercise can be made a lot more difficult by doing it with your eyes closed, but make sure that you are standing next to something you can hold onto in case you get wobbly.

The following daily foot exercises will help strengthen your feet and speed up your progress:

Toe Squeezes – Squeeze your toes together as firmly as you can and hold for a few seconds. Relax for a couple of seconds and repeat. Do two sets of twelve repetitions with each foot.

Toe spreads – Spread your toes as far and wide apart as you can by using your toe muscles. In other words, flare them sideways. Hold this position for a few seconds, then relax. Do two sets of twelve repetitions per foot.

Foot pointers – Point your toes firmly towards the floor in front of you and hold the position for a few seconds. Then point your toes the opposite way towards your face and hold for a few seconds. Repeat the process twelve times with each foot.

Foot rolls – Sit on the floor, bend your left knee, and grab hold of the sides of your left foot with both hands. Use your hands to lever the foot, turning it outwards and inwards, giving it a good pull in both directions. Repeat twelve times on each foot.

6. Barefoot sports and activities. Within a few weeks of starting, most people will be able to get to the final stage, which is living the barefoot lifestyle. What I mean by this is that you are either barefoot or wearing minimal shoes for the majority of your days, regardless of what activity you are doing. With the correct technique, there is a natural progression from barefoot walking to barefoot running, golf, tennis, bowls, and hockey. In fact, most sports are possible to participate in while wearing minimal footwear. When you reach this stage, your foot will continue to strengthen, and you will continue to reap the benefits of your hard work with fewer injuries and much-improved performance in your chosen sport due to enhanced foot sense and overall kinesthetic sense, body balance, function, and a better posture.

SHARON'S UNWINDING STORY

English Teacher, 60

I've suffered from extremely flat feet and turned-in knees since I was very young. After a lifetime of suffering, it was finally decided, fourteen years ago, that surgery was the best option to help my feet. Unfortunately, the nerves in my feet were disturbed during the operation, and I was left with numbness in my feet, which I was told would be permanent. This affected my balance (I used to topple over when leaning forwards or bending) and I was only able to walk short distances. Sometimes I needed crutches to get out of bed in the mornings. My feet were constantly cold due to poor circulation and my legs were often puffy. Standing for long periods resulted in backache, as I tended to shift my weight to my left side.

I started my ABC™ treatment in May 2018, and since then, everything has changed. I now have recovered full feeling in my feet, which has given me back my balance. My crutches are now obsolete; I no longer need them at all. I can walk without pain, my posture is vastly improved, and I'm able to enjoy things I haven't done for fourteen years. Being able to be more active is also helping me lose weight. Other people are also noticing a change in the way that I carry myself, which is helping with my confidence. I enjoy my weekly session and continue to make improvements. To anyone who is thinking of trying structural correction, all I can say is, "Book your appointment now!" They have improved my life and wellbeing far more than I ever could have expected or hoped.

CHAPTER 7

Sleeping Well

"Sleep is the golden chain that ties health and our bodies together."

—*Thomas Dekker*

There are few things as important to your health as a good night's sleep. Yet, it is an area in which many people struggle, whether they aren't able to fall asleep, wake up frequently, experience neck and back pain while in bed, or simply don't get good enough quality sleep to wake up feeling refreshed.

Poor sleep has been linked to chronic pain, obesity, cancer, lowered immunity, anxiety, heart disease, and essentially every serious chronic health problem we face. When you sleep, your body regenerates and resets itself, readying itself to fight another day. If your sleep is consistently cut short or is of insufficient quality, the sleep deprivation that ensues can leave you locked in a vicious cycle of high stress and under-recovery.

Prioritising and optimising sleep should be extremely high on your health agenda, but for many people it simply is not. I think the reason for this is that sleep suffers from an image crisis; it is simply not sexy to focus on going to bed early or staying in bed long enough to properly recover and renew from the stresses of the previous day. Modern society has created conditions whereby it is far more attractive to be seen as someone who gets a lot done. Getting up at the crack of dawn and staying up late to work and produce like a superhero is glorified.

I am all for being highly productive and doing what is required to get ahead in life, but not when it comes at the expense of my health. I have seen far too many people's worlds fall apart after they lost their health. There is so often an attitude of "It will never happen to me" or "One day, when I get further ahead, I will take care of my health and catch up." The problem is that good, hard-working people *do* experience health crises out of the blue. If you aren't willing to put your health first today, what makes you think that you will in the future? The best time will always be now, and good sleep is most definitely one of the small levers that swings a big door.

There are two aspects of sleeping well. The first is quantity. There's no need to draw this topic out, but at a minimum, you must get the required seven to nine hours of sleep per night. The simplest way to achieve that is to go to bed at the same time every night and wake up at the same time each morning. Having this set routine is important because it trains your internal body clock, known as your circadian rhythm, back into balance. All of your internal organs and body systems are regulated by your circadian rhythm. It ties in with every biological process from digestion to hormones to metabolism. The sad fact, which is backed up by science, is that most people in the Western world have a chronically disrupted circadian rhythm. This does not bode well in their quest for a high-energy, high-performing, healthy, and pain-free body! The simplest way to reset this rhythm is through a sleep schedule, which has the added bonus of ensuring that you get enough sleep.

Remember the old adage that "hours before midnight count as two?" Our body clocks are synched to the natural rhythm of nature, which is set by the rise and fall of the sun. So, ideally, the sooner after sunset that you are asleep, the better. It is wise to try to be in bed by 9:30pm and asleep by 10:30pm, at the latest. If you want proof as to the importance of your circadian rhythms, look no further than the numerous studies done on shift workers, who have been shown to have an increased risk of certain cancers as well as metabolic problems, heart disease, ulcers, gastrointestinal problems, and obesity.

The second crucial aspect of sleep is quality, which essentially speaks to how well you sleep. Not all sleep is created equal. The only way that you will know if you are sleeping through the night and getting the appropriate amount of deep, restful sleep versus waking up frequently with restless sleep is to track it. There are several good sleep tracking devices and apps on the market that can help you quantify just how well you are sleeping. It is well worth it to invest in one of these so that you can take a look at real data and objectively see how well you are doing. The added bonus is that when you measure something, it generally tends to improve.

It is common for people to toss and turn as well as wake up frequently throughout the night. There are many reasons why this happens, including a high emotional stress load, blood sugar problems, electromagnetic radiation, being exposed to too much blue light in the evening (by staring at computer screens, TV's, tablets, and mobile phones), a too-high room temperature, or a room that's not completely dark. Even the five lumens of light that are emitted from a small LED on an electrical device in the corner of your room have been demonstrated through research to cause disruption to one's circadian rhythm. Your room needs to be pitch black—so black, in fact, that you can't see your hand in front of your face. If you struggle to create these conditions with blackout blinds, get one of the several good sleep masks on the market. There are several factors to consider when it comes to high-quality sleep, and I've only broached some of the common ones. You should definitely address those, but they aren't where I want to place the greatest focus. There is another commonly overlooked and misunderstood factor that can make the biggest difference of all to the quality of your sleep, and that is how you support your skeletal frame in bed.

If your back and neck cannot relax completely as you lie down, your nervous system will be forced into defence physiology. Muscles will have to contract in order to stabilise the problematically misaligned vertebrae, and that structural tension—combined with the stretch on your meninges, brain, and spinal cord—can make it impossible to "switch off" to the degree required to sleep soundly through the night. With your brain and body on guard, you will toss and turn, endlessly trying to find a position where your body can let go and rest.

If you regularly experience restless nights and wake up frequently; it takes you a long time to drift off; or your neck, back, or hips ache when you are in bed and you wake up with the pillow on the other side of the room, the duvet turned inside out, and your head on the opposite corner of the bed where the cat usually sleeps, it is highly likely that something is wrong with your mattress, pillow, or sleeping position. Oftentimes, all three. Similarly, if you wake up in the morning and creak on your way to the bathroom even though you felt fine the evening before, please don't ignore that feedback from your body. You are not simply getting older, and this is not what you have to put up with from now on. This is evidence that your musculoskeletal system is locked up tightly in a compensation pattern that was trying to stabilise your body throughout the night. Remember, if it looks like a duck, walks like a duck, and quacks like a duck, it's not a zebra. It's a duck. Far too often, I see people overlook the simple and obvious feedback their bodies give them. If you don't want to hear your body scream, listen to it when it whispers. Pay attention to and fix the most obvious and likely problems first.

There are many different possibilities to consider when it comes to why you could be sleeping poorly. Getting the right mattress and pillow is part of the twenty percent of habits that can give you eighty percent of the results that you seek. They are often done poorly, so there is a lot to gain from doing them properly. An added benefit of high-quality sleep—besides enhanced recovery from stress and improved energy and overall health stats—is that your structural health can stabilise. If you are allowing your back and body joints to relax properly through the night without perpetually creating new problems, you will find a much more stable balance point in your body and reap the rewards of greater strength and resilience through the rest of your life.

CHOOSING THE RIGHT MATTRESS

When your body has bones out of place in a direction from which they cannot self-correct, they are not just stuck forwards. They are stuck forwards *and* twisted to the side. On top of this gets layered the tensioning effect of the compensation pattern, and your body ends up twisted in multiple directions in three dimensions.

When your body finds itself in this sort of condition, the only way you can get comfortable is to have a mattress that is soft enough to allow you to twist in three dimensions whilst taking pressure off as many areas as possible. Unfortunately, the same positions that allow you to get the most comfortable are also those that force the body further into its misalignment pattern. When you get your body corrected with ABC™ so that your entire structure lines up correctly, the twist comes out and muscles no longer pull in directions that they shouldn't. The twisting effect becomes greatly reduced, and with the improved alignment and flexibility it becomes important to provide enough support to your structure when resting to keep it that way. It needs a very firm mattress that prevents you from sinking into it and twisting.

This is sometimes a difficult concept to learn and can involve some trial and error. Usually, when patients first begin treatment, their bodies are so twisted up that the only mattress they can get comfortable on is a soft one (on which they've spent a lot of money). A few weeks into care, they typically begin complaining of waking up feeling stiff and sore in their lower back or elsewhere. This is not actually a problem; it is a sign of progress. Now that their body mechanics have improved and sufficiently unlocked, they have progressed to a level where more support is needed in order to maintain healthy alignment through the night.

The worst sort of mattress is one that uses memory foam. Unfortunately, these are commonly purchased given the effective marketing tactics of their parent companies. However, they are far too yielding and will quickly cause a person's care to plateau. They won't make further progress until they switch to something firmer. There are a great number of mattresses available to try, and thankfully many companies offer a trial period. If you don't like it, you can send it back. I recommend beginning with the firmest pocket-sprung mattress you can find. If it is too much to tolerate in the beginning because you get pressure sores on your hips or shoulders, you can add a one-inch topper for a while until you improve enough mechanically to easily tolerate the firmness. This usually solves the problem while still giving your body the support that is needed. As your body mechanics improve, you will be able to remove the topper and have the next level of firmness readily available. The advanced solution for people who are further down the road with their structural correction or are mechanically healthy enough to stand it is to sleep on a 5 - 8cm latex topper placed on top of a flat wooden board. This provides the appropriate amount of support for the healthiest of spines, and also enough comfort that you will still enjoy sleeping.

Some people like to use futons or even Japanese tatami mats, although these are very firm, and it may take months or even years before you progress to the point that you can sleep well on them.

CHOOSING THE RIGHT PILLOW

There is a dizzying array of pillow options out there. Should you go for on that's feather-filled or made of memory foam? The firm one or the soft one? Should it be flat, curved, dimpled, or contoured? What about the one that keeps showing up on the adverts? Also, should you be using said pillow while lying on your front, back, or side? Do you need another one between your knees? It's all quite confusing, and I'll explain to you why this confusion exists.

The first problem is that pillow manufacturers market their pillows with the idea that somehow the neck should be lifted into a "neutral" position such that the head and neck line up with the spine.

Interestingly, much of the research I have read on the effects of pillow height on neck and back health was conducted with this basis as well, but is it correct? The answer becomes clear when you consider all the complicated ways in which a person's spine can be misaligned. By this point, you are vividly aware that bones misalign forwards and the spine compensates by tilting and twisting, leading to a twisted, three-dimensional configuration unique to each person. This means that in order to support the spine, you need to line it up and support the head and neck according to the way the spine *actually is* in present reality, not how it *should be* in some ideal anatomical scenario.

This point makes all the difference in the world when it comes to getting quality sleep all the way through the night. Remember that when you are sleeping, you are not dead. You are simply in a lowered state of awareness, but your brain is still sensing your environment. The quality of your sleep and how rested you feel in the morning comes down to whether or not you can find and maintain a comfortable position throughout the night. If you become uncomfortable at any point, you will shift around, perhaps even waking up to move until you find comfort. The more that you move during the night, the less rest you will get. It's that simple.

Consider what happens when you use a soft pillow such as a feather pillow. You fluff it up or punch it down so that it is the right height to allow you to get comfortable and fall asleep. During the night, it is quite likely that the pillow will change height, causing your body to twist, turn, or bend, eventually causing discomfort. Therefore, you'll move in your sleep or wake up and purposefully move in order to get comfortable again. Regardless, the quality of your sleep has been reduced and you may wake up with stiff and achy back, neck, or shoulders. You may even have a headache.

Another scenario is, you arrange a pillow into what feels like a comfortable position, and you fall asleep. However, the position is not correct for your spine and it puts a twist, turn, or bend into your spine that becomes uncomfortable, causing you to move or wake up and move. Again, the more often you need to move, the less restful your sleep will be, and the more uncomfortable you may be in the morning.

Pain and discomfort mainly occur at points in your body that have been under prolonged twisting tension (remember the discussion on compensations in Chapter 4). If you are doubting this, try this very simple experiment.

EXPERIMENT

Grab the end of your left thumb with you right thumb and index finger. Keeping your left-hand position steady, turn your left thumb joint clockwise as far as it goes. You will notice a twisting tension form through the thumb joint itself. Keep that twisting tension on for a few minutes (when you have some idle time) and you will notice that it gradually gets more and more uncomfortable. You can even have another person squeeze the knuckle joint of your thumb as you maintain this twist and you will see that the joint itself is now very tender and painful. Let go of the twist and you will experience an immediate relief, and if you squeeze the thumb joint again you will notice that all pain and tenderness has now gone.

We are left with the reality that achieving a quality night's sleep and feeling comfortable and flexible in our body in the morning comes down to how successfully you find and maintain a stable position throughout the night. This is why there are so many different pillows on the market. There are so many different shapes and sizes of bodies as well as ways that a body can become misaligned, making the discovery of that "perfect position" of comfort quite challenging. This is why people commonly spend a small fortune testing out pillows until they find one that they like. At which point, they will defend that pillow to the death and cling to it for the rest of time.

You don't need to go down that expensive road or have an unhealthy attachment to the only pillow you love. Fortunately, there is a consistent and predictable method for building your own pillow at the perfect height for your spine, regardless of whether you are at home or on holiday. With this method, you will be able to get comfortable and stay comfortable all night long. When you get it right, you'll be amazed because not only will you fall asleep quickly, you'll wake up in the exact same position, feeling refreshed and ready to go.

THE WORST POSITION TO SLEEP IN

For as long as they have existed doctors and chiropractors have been advising people *not* to sleep on their fronts. Most front-sleepers know this, yet they cannot stop themselves from doing it.

Humour me for a minute; I've got another experiment for you to try. Sit upright and turn your head to the left as far as it will go; now turn it just a little bit further. Good. Now, I'll see you in eight hours! Obviously, this is not going to be enjoyable for you or your neck, so if you don't finish the experiment, I won't hold it against you. But do spare a thought for your neck joints and muscles if you are a front sleeper. They are being put under a lot of unnecessary strain.

Whilst a neck can turn to eighty or ninety degrees, it is not meant to stay there for long periods of time. Sleeping on your front risks the development or further aggravation of headaches, neck pain, back pain, shoulder pain, or arm pain. It is likely that your sleep quality will be reduced as well, which (as we've discussed) has further reaching consequences than just your joints and muscles.

When I was eight years old, my mum took me to see the local chiropractor. Fortunately for my future career ambitions, she has always been open-minded and willing to test things out in order to discover what works best. Upon discovering that I was a front sleeper, this chiropractor gave us some quite creative advice to solve the problem. He advised us to buy some sewing elastic and cut it to a length that would fit snugly around my abdomen. His next suggestion was to get three plastic hair rollers (the round, spiky tubes that used to be all the rage in the eighties. I've no idea if they even still make these!). I was advised to thread them through the elastic so that they were loosely held into position on the front of my abdomen, ready and waiting to spike should I roll onto my front. I don't ever remember waking up as a result of setting off the trap, but I do remember that from the very first night of wearing that contraption, I never again slept on my front.

The reason I tell this story is that front sleepers will often fiercely defend their sleeping position, claiming it to be super comfortable (or declaring the inability to stop themselves from doing it). I'm not saying that it's easy to avoid sleeping on your front, but if you set the intention of breaking the habit, you can absolutely do it. If you are a front sleeper, it is advised that you do whatever it takes to figure out another way to get through the night. Here are the recommended alternatives:

THE BACK-SLEEPING OPTION

Sleeping on your back is perfectly acceptable and an easy position in which to get comfortable, but it is important that you get your pillow height correct. The most common mistake back sleepers make is using a pillow that is too high, which pushes the head forwards and aggravates or creates problems by levering the lower neck and upper back vertebrae forwards.

Remember, forwards-stuck vertebrae are not a good thing because your body cannot pull them back. When you wake up in the morning, you will need to compensate by tilting your neck into extension, leading to a stiff and painful neck, back, and shoulders. This is a common mistake and one with huge long-term consequences. I have seen many patients slow to respond to care or with persistent Dowager's Humps suddenly make rapid progress when this problem was discovered and addressed. Sleeping on your back with a pillow that is too high can create posture problems every time you sleep, a fact easily understood by paying attention to your own body (and not surprisingly shown to be true through research). The higher the pillow, the greater the mechanical strain placed on your neck.[35] The first goal is to sleep through the night; the second is to do so without stressing, straining, or misaligning your spine.

Your spine needs to be in as neutral a position as possible in order to relax. This means that if you sleep on your back, your head needs to be nearly flat for the spine to align correctly—a position that becomes impossible to achieve with almost every commercially available pillow. This essential element of biomechanics appears to be poorly understood, even by researchers. Most of the studies available look only at different types of pillows, and the ones that explore pillow height neglect to compare against the mechanically correct neutral position. The reason for this is likely that locked-forwards head postures are so common these days that most people are uncomfortable lying on their back *without* a pillow. The meninges become so scarred and taught in an effort to protect the multiple forwards-stuck bones that they don't allow for natural extension to easily occur.

This common degenerative posture problem, which we call a hard kyphosis (essentially an upper back/neck that is curved and stuck too far forwards) can be corrected almost immediately with the ABC™ method, and I demonstrate it to patients on an almost daily basis. I first have the person with kyphosis lie on the floor and notice how their back bends. Usually, the mid-back is so curved and stiff that the head has to extend significantly in order to reach the floor. In some cases, it does not reach the floor at all; it's simply stuck in the air. I then lie them on the adjusting table and carry out what is called the Anterior Meningeal Release, which is a skilled manual stretching procedure that breaks up adhesions within the meninges. I then have the patient lie back down on the floor, and they are often pleasantly surprised by how much their mid-back has relaxed and how easily they are able get their head on the floor without tension. In more advanced cases, it may take a few sessions to loosen completely, but it *is* possible to unlock those hard kyphosis postures and get people comfortable on their backs once again.

Correcting this sort of problem is essential to good health. If you remember back to Chapter 2, it was noted that people who have bodies with hard kyphosis have a strong correlation with heart disease and die at a greater rate than the non-kyphotic population.

BUILDING YOUR PERFECT PILLOW: IF YOU SLEEP ON YOUR BACK

Here's the part you've been waiting for: the simple method for designing a pillow that fits and supports your unique body. If you're a back sleeper, the process is simple. Take a small towel, fold it in half, take one end and fold it again to meet the middle (halfway) point of the towel. This will create a stepped pillow whereby half of it is two layers deep and the other half is four layers deep. (See Figure 9).

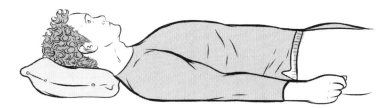

[Figure 9A] A standing pillow is too high pushing the head and neck forwards

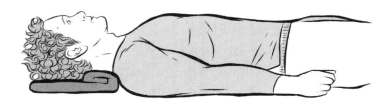

[Figure 9B] Folded towels to the correct height allow the neck to rest in good alignment

Your head rests on the thinner layer, and the thicker layer goes under your neck. You should only feel a slight touch of the towel on your neck. If you feel it pushing your neck up, the towels are too high. Start again with a thinner towel until you get it right.

If you are used to sleeping on your back with a big pillow under your head, this will feel weird at first. It will feel too low. That's ok; trust the process and pay attention to how your spine feels. You should notice that it is relaxed and not under any stress or strain.

Remember that if your pillow is too high when you lie on your back, you may well feel comfortable in the moment, but it puts a forwards pressure on your vertebrae, making it likely that you will get neck or back pain or tension during the night or when you wake up in the morning.

If you have a hard kyphotic posture (where your back curves forwards more than normal), it can be quite uncomfortable to lie flat, so a very thin pillow on top of the towels may work to provide adequate support to your neck. However, if you have a stooped posture, you will find it easier to perfect your pillow situation in the side-lying position, which is the most ideal option.

BUILDING YOUR PERFECT PILLOW: THE SIDE-SLEEPING OPTION

This is the best position for getting comfortable and properly supporting your spine, but it does require you to get your pillow height exactly right. We have found through experimentation over the years that the difference in size between a pillow that is "just right" and a pillow that is "dead wrong" (which is any height other than "just right"), can be as little as 1-2 mm. That may seem like an exaggeration, but it's truth will become clear when you test this method for yourself.

There is currently no commercial pillow available that allows you to adjust its height to this degree of specificity, so once again towels come to the rescue. All you do is continue to add or remove layers of towels until you find the perfect fit for your body. Start with a couple of folded towels that are roughly the height of the distance between your shoulder and where it meets the base of your neck; then test it out by lying on your side and following these simple rules:

Rule 1: If it is too low, you will feel your body rolling forwards, so add another single layer of towel and test it again.

Rule 2: If it is too high, you will feel your body moving backwards, so remove a layer of towel and test again.

Keep going until you find the balanced midpoint, which is precisely where you need to be. You will know when you have found it because your body will feel still and there will be no tension in your spine. Oftentimes, your eyes will also feel heavy and want to close within about thirty seconds of being in this "perfect position." (See Figure 10).

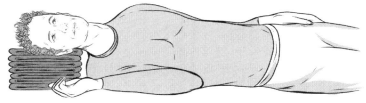

[Figure 10A] Pillow is too high and the body pushes backwards

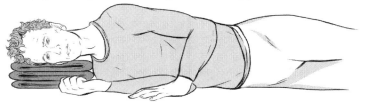

[Figure 10B] Pillow is too low and the body falls forwards

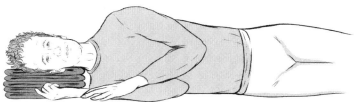

[Figure 10C] Pillow height is correct and the body remains relaxed and perfectly balanced

What you will notice is that even one layer of towel makes a difference. This is a great way to discover once and for all that your spine is a precision instrument that needs to be precisely supported in order to be able to relax. It can take ten to twenty minutes of testing to find the perfect height, so be patient and keep going until you get it right! When you find the perfect fit, put a pillowcase over the towels to prevent them from getting ruffled up or moving during the night.

If you travel a lot, ask the hotel to provide extra towels because you can almost guarantee that a hotel bed and pillow combination will drive you crazy, especially if you're getting corrected with ABC™ and your body is craving more support.

There is also a special ABC™ pillow which is available to purchase through most practitioners. It is made from lots of different-sized sections of foam that make it easy and more practical to find the perfect height for your body.

PAULA'S UNWINDING STORY

English Teacher, 57

Omg! This works. Thank you so much. Yesterday, looking at the state of the four pillows on my bed I decided that they needed to be changed. I was about to buy new ones when I remembered the advice you give for the foam pillows or the homemade towel version. It's so typical of me to have disregarded it as I have a lung condition and experience breathing issues at night, so I convinced myself I needed four pillows.

I gave it a go replaced four pillows with four towels. I have just woken from the best night's sleep in years—no headache, no neck ache, no pins and needles in my arm, and I slept through the night (I normally wake up three or four times). Brilliant. Thank you, Richard, and the whole team. You also taught me to stop being so set in my ways in future. I'll be drinking kale smoothies next.

CHAPTER 8

Sitting Well

"Sitting is the new smoking."

—*Unknown*

If you were designing a way to secretly and efficiently ruin a human body, you would be hard-pressed to invent a product more devastating than the humble four-legged chair. Flying under the radar for generations, this simple modern invention has wreaked untold havoc on the human frame, and it wasn't until recently that the true extent of the impact of sitting has become a known concern.

Since this information has recently hit the mainstream media, you may have heard sitting referred to as the "new smoking." Recent research has revealed concerning details about the devastating impact of this seemingly innocuous activity, leading one author, Dr. James Levine, also a Mayo Clinic director, to take it a few steps further and say that, "Sitting is more dangerous than smoking, kills more people than HIV, and is more treacherous than parachuting." He sums up his thoughts in one crisp sentence, "We are sitting ourselves to death".[36]

Australian researchers have also suggested that sitting is more harmful than smoking, explaining that for every hour that you watch television after the age of twenty-five, your life expectancy decreases by 21.8 minutes.[37] By comparison, smoking a single cigarette reduces one's life expectancy by an estimated eleven minutes.[38] When put into that context, alarm bells start to ring, and we can begin recognising the need for a significant change in terms of our approach to this activity.

There is a mountain of evidence and expert opinions (and it's growing) that shows that sitting is not only harmful to the human frame, it's also bad for general health. It may come as a surprise that sitting for just two consecutive hours can increase the risk of heart disease, diabetes, metabolic syndrome, and cancer as well as back pain, neck pain, and many other orthopaedic problems.[39] To put the impact of a sedentary lifestyle into perspective, the World Health Organisation has ranked physical inactivity (sitting too much) as the fourth biggest preventable killer globally, killing more than 3.2 million people a year.[40]

While information like this is not to be taken lightly, it also doesn't make solving the root cause of the problem easy because so many of us are working jobs that require long periods of sitting throughout the day. This has caused a slow, insidious decline in our structural health, resulting in office workers experiencing more musculoskeletal injuries than industry sector workers in industries such as construction, transport, and metal. Sitting has become as much of an occupational risk as heavy lifting.[41] Personally, I am convinced that sitting for long periods of time is the most significant burden people place on their bodies. It has greatly contributed to the structural decline of modern man, and it has done so almost completely under the radar. We never saw this epidemic coming!

Sitting is yet another example of a man-made modern stressor that is working against biology. Our evolutionary environment was very different from today's conditions, yet the routines of the past are what forged our genetics and engineered our human machine. For much of the last two million years of evolution, the human body has been walking (evidence suggests that our hunter-gatherer ancestors walked as much as a marathon distance every day), running, sleeping, leaning, foraging, and squatting—doing the things that kept them alive. It sounds like very hard work these days, but all of those millennia spent surviving literally forged the human design. We evolved while spending the majority of our time on the move, and this is what our nervous systems expect based upon our biology. A symbiotic relationship has evolved between our movement patterns and our health. We are built to move, and movement keeps us healthy.

The chair, in contrast, is a relatively recent addition to the timeline of human existence. It's only been around for some five hundred generations or so. In the beginning, a chair was simply a place to rest a weary body after a day spent in the fields or factory. Furniture likely had a minimal impact on body structure in these early days, but fast-forward to today, and in a time span of around fifty years we have become almost completely sedentary beings.

The sedentary lifestyle that chairs have afforded us is a new and unique structural stress to which we have been exposed for a relatively short period of time in the grand scheme of things. Unfortunately, evolution does not have foresight, which means that genes forged long ago are poorly matched with the reality of modern lifestyles. This means that we are only just now starting to understand the impact of the movement deficiency syndrome that has befallen modern man. Equally, we have not had enough time for our physical design to evolve and meet these new demands. As a result, a slumped and degenerated human frame is now almost pandemic throughout society, with huge consequences on both physical and mental health and performance.

If you were to sit for just ten minutes with good form, on a healthy chair, the effects would be easily tolerated by your body. The difficulty with sitting is the same as the difficulty with junk food: it's difficult to stop after eating just one square of chocolate. Generally, the whole bar is going down. As well, we don't do just a little bit of sitting; we do a lot. The average British person sits for seven to nine hours per day, and as one research poll suggested, Brits spend more time sitting on the toilet each week than they do exercising.[42]

You may consider yourself an active individual. Perhaps you go to the gym or play a sport for an hour a day and think that this is undoing or somehow making up for the fact that you spend the rest of your day parked behind a desk. Unfortunately, that's not the case. Alarmingly, studies have shown that the negative effects of long-term sitting are not reversible through exercise or other good habits. You may want to read that last sentence again. The first time I read the research, I was quite surprised because it really brings into perspective the enormous impact of modern lifestyles. This evidence means that you can eat the perfect diet, do your dutiful one hour in the gym, meditate before and after work, and pray to the heavens for good health, but if you sit for much of your remaining waking hours of the day, the stress placed on your system will be enough to cancel out all the other good work that you did to support your health.[43] It's a good example of an inconvenient truth, but it can also be a motivating poke in the ribs.

Wake-up calls are often uncomfortable, but if you truly want to live in the rare air with a healthy, fully functioning body, you will start to make different choices. It's funny to think just how much of our lives are lived on autopilot. Once we get used to an action, it becomes a habit and is stored in the subconscious mind requiring next to no effort to maintain. The same goes for both the good and the bad habits you form. Once you start to question your daily habits, you can begin to replace the harmful ones with healthier actions. Once those actions become a habit, you will have literally changed the trajectory of the rest of your life. Remember, you become your habits. If you want to predict your future, just look at how you live today. One of my favourite sayings is, "Your days are your life in miniature." Thank you for that, Robin Sharma. It says it all.

The rude truth that an hour at the gym cannot and will not protect you from the ill effects of excessive sitting should not come as a surprise at this point. There are two basic issues that general exercise will not address. The first is the mechanical problems created by sitting. Excess time spent in modern furniture forces your spine into a curve and locks the bones forwards in positions that cannot be reversed. No amount of stretching, strengthening, or moving will realign those bones and correct the resulting underling mechanical problems. The forwards-slumped posture and stretching of the spinal cord and brainstem that occur as a result can have harmful, long-term effects on both structural and neurological health. Sitting, in effect, sets up a runaway train of dysfunction in your body that can eventually lead to multiple debilitating problems with pain, injury, fatigue, loss of performance, and all manner of other organ-related issues, many of which we covered extensively in Chapter 2, Alignment Matters.

Structural problems are unfortunately a self-fulfilling reality because if your body is hurting or you lose trust in it, expecting it to fail on you based on your past experiences, you'll be far less likely to move enough to create good health. Being able to trust your body to handle the rigours of life, sport, and exercise is an important factor driving the desire to be active and the intensity with which you approach it. High performers develop an implicit trust that their bodies will support them no matter what conditions they face. Having that kind of strong foundation is one of the great secrets of world class performers in any field—as the saying goes, "As in body, so in mind."

That cycle of dysfunction must be broken, and fortunately, the problems caused by sitting can be reduced by improving on your choice of chairs and making a few adjustments to the way you park your bum in them. I'm going to teach you the few simple tweaks that go a long way in this area. But, unfortunately, even if you manage to mitigate the damaging biomechanical impact of sitting, there is still the elephant in the room to deal with, which is that you are not moving your body enough overall if you sit for a living. Multiple hours of sitting create a deficiency in movement that cannot simply be made up for with a furious hour of exercise.

You are hard-wired to move, and movement tunes your physiology, so you have to figure out how to give your body more of what it needs. This is such a simple discussion when it comes to nutrition. If your levels of vitamin C got low enough, for example, you will develop a nasty condition called scurvy. If you run low enough on vitamin B1, you will suffer from a condition called beriberi. A vitamin B12 deficiency can lead to anaemia, amongst other issues. The solutions are usually simple: just eat more of the foods that contain these nutrients. These conditions don't spontaneously develop; they are created through a lack of something. The broader truth is that illness can only exist when health is lacking.

Consider that movement works in the same way, much like an essential nutrient you need to consume in order to function normally. Movement impacts every single system and part of your body. Take only your brain, as an example, on which we have learned that movement works in much the same way as does fertiliser on a field. Exercise leads to the production of a growth factor called brain-derived neurotrophic factor (BDNF). BDNF allows us to make new synaptic connections in our brains and learn new material. This process is called neurogenesis, and it is crucial for the developing brain in childhood as well as the slowing of the natural aging process later in life. In order to think well, you must be moving well, which creates a strong case against the use of chairs in schools and offices, or at the very least, support of limiting their use. Our brains simply do not perform at their best when we are sedentary.

So, what can you do to avoid this sort of burden on your body? The first step is to change or adapt your furniture so that it doesn't harm your body mechanics and posture. The next step is to limit the amount of time that you spend sitting, even if you have adapted your chairs to be less damaging. This requires becoming more active throughout the day (and I'm not referring to adding in one hour of exercise over lunch time. That's not enough).

ENDING THE CURSE OF MODERN FURNITURE

The problem that needs to be solved with many seats, chairs, and sofas is the way that they force your body into a forwards curve. They are designed like this in order to accommodate modern-day poor postures, but whilst they may be more comfortable for a forwards-stuck body, they are also a trap. Every moment you spend relaxing in that position is perpetuating the problem. If you want to rebuild an upright body, it becomes imperative that you choose seating options that encourage good alignment and postures rather than accommodate poor ones.

Just as with poor shoes and soft mattresses, if patients undergoing structural correction sit in the wrong chairs, it is very difficult to correct their body mechanics. New problems are created just as quickly as the old ones were cleared out. Fortunately, this can be overcome, but it must be taken seriously. Nature does not bend to your choices, she simply adapts to the stress, and the end result is is always a problem-riddled body.

Let's get into some specifics. The big issue with many chairs, even the high-tech, ergonomic, £1000 one, is that they dip down at the back, positioning your buttocks lower than your legs. That is the key piece to understand.

THE STRAIGHT TRUTH

If, when you sit, your thighs angle downwards towards your hips, your spine will be forced forwards.

This is common even on hard, wooden chairs, but especially when it comes to just about every chair that is cushioned. Sofas are particularly harmful in this regard, and I have not found a single sofa over years of testing many different styles and designs that has not forced my body into a poor posture. There is a way to take a sofa and make it even worse, and that is by turning it into a recliner (or a *decliner*, as I have heard them called by ABC™ practitioners describing their health degrading effects). Sitting in these soft chairs and reclining backwards reverses the natural curves of your spine and significantly worsens your mechanics, so these types of chairs are especially worth avoiding.

Have you ever noticed that friends or family members will sit on sofas in some pretty peculiar postures? Folding one or both legs under or twisting and leaning heavily to one side? What's happening here is, their body is trying to add in tension (compensate) in order to find stability because the base is too soft, and their spine is being pushed forwards. This is very often the reason people prefer to sit cross-legged or lean back on their chair; it makes it easier to compensate for their mechanical problems. It should highlight for you, however, that the chair is inadequate for their needs. If you get adjusted with ABC™ and then sit on a chair that supports you properly, you will not feel the need to cross your legs or fidget. Your body will settle into a restful neutral position and can remain there for hours without bothering you. When your spine is correctly aligned, it has proper leverage and can effortlessly resist gravity.

Car seats are arguably the worst offenders of them all, designed out of necessity into a bucket shape in order to fit a human being into the car. They would have to significantly increase the roof height of cars in order to create a better seating arrangement, which is clearly unlikely to happen. Instead, bodies have to bend in order to fit. Often the "bananafication" effect of sitting in a car seat is made worse by a headrest that angles forwards. Yet another example of modern design accommodating dysfunctional bodies. If you are stuck forwards and the headrest is not configured forwards, you will be uncomfortable and straining as you drive. But, if your body is healthy and upright (or at least not significantly degenerated forwards) this one seemingly small adjustment could cause problems by forcing your head and neck forwards. You probably already know that your car seat is not good for you, since it is unlikely that you jump out of it feeling like a spring chicken. Even just ten minutes in the car can leave you feeling locked up and tired. Imagine spending ten hours per week in one, being bananafied! That is the average amount of time spent per week in the car in the UK, by the way. Remember, any time you have difficulty getting out of a chair of any sort and find it challenging to straighten up and walk away feeling loose, your body was just made worse by that chair. No excuses. No stories. No justifications. That's the mechanical reality of human bodies pitted against chairs. If you learn to pay attention to those biological feedback cues, you can figure your way through the maddening maze that is modern furniture.

THE SIMPLE FIX FOR MOST CHAIRS

Yesterday, as I had lunch in a local cafe, I observed a gentleman sitting opposite me, eating his soup. I couldn't help but notice that he was in an extremely stooped position, with his spine curved into a hyperkyphosis and his neck angled sharply backwards. The most interesting moment to watch was the one in which he stood up. He maintained that same forwards-stuck posture, only his legs and pelvis tilted and twisted to allow him to remain upright (the compensation pattern). He looked like a human question-mark, and he was a relatively young man, no older than forty, I would guess. His body had become literally locked into an aged position. As I watched him leave, I thought about how much of an impact this poor posture would have on his life. Ironically, he is probably largely unaware that he has an underlying mechanical problem, since not everyone with poor posture has pain. He has probably been told to straighten up numerous times, but since he can't maintain that position with effort alone, he likely gave up trying to sort out his posture years ago. Once a new "normal" settles in, we so easily forget what full function feels like—how it feels to take a deep, unrestricted breath; how it feels to move, bend, and lift effortlessly; what it feels like to wake up and go to bed feeling loose and agile. The rediscovering of these lost functions is one of the most fun things to witness as clients go through structural correction. It's curious, but not only do we not know what we don't know, we quickly forget how we used to feel and easily settle into new dynamics. As I reflected further, a sadder fact was the likely scenario that his body had got this way from years and years of making the same basic errors of sitting on the wrong chairs for far too long, simply because he didn't and doesn't know what he didn't and doesn't know.

Here is what you need to be aware about when it comes to chairs: the single biggest problem that needs to be fixed is the dip at the back of the chair, where your buttocks go. This dip is present on nearly all chairs, including car seats, sofas, high-tech office chairs, reception chairs, restaurant chairs, and airplane seats. If it has four legs supporting a flat surface, chances are it dips down at the back.

Remember that this is a problem because when your buttocks sinks lower than your knees, your body will stoop and suffer.

Fortunately, you can improve most chairs with the simple addition of a foam seat wedge. This is something that I recommend everybody place on their chairs, because they will tilt your pelvis forwards slightly (or in the case of a very soft or deep chair, at least give you a more level surface to work with) into a healthier position for your body. Doing this improves the natural leverage that you have over your spine in the same way that using a heel chip does in your shoes. It also provides your spine with a firm, supportive structure to rest on, stopping it from sinking into the chair's cushioned surface. Obviously, there is a limit as to how soft a chair can be to begin with before a seat wedge isn't even helpful, which is why most sofas will forever be a problem. Nevertheless, place a seat wedge on every surface that you sit, and you will immediately reduce the burden that gravity places on your spine.

Making this one simple change can have a big impact, and many people are surprised by how much better they feel when they sit this way. Typically, people report feeling a lot less tired and achy at the end of the day. (See Figure 11)

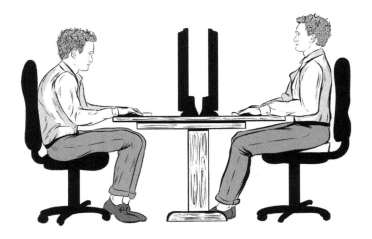

[**Figure 11**] Without a seat wedge the pelvis sinks down into the chair causing posture to fail forwards.

Using a seat wedge lifts the pelvis up and angles the thighs downwards, encouraging a relaxed upright posture.

TIPS FOR MAKING BETTER SITTING AND RESTING CHOICES

Here are some changes to consider making to your seating arrangements at home and work:

1. An ideal chair has a completely flat and firm surface to sit on. Ideally, you are able to tilt this surface forward about ten degrees to allow the pelvis to tilt forward and position your hips above your knees so that your thighs slope downwards towards the floor. Some of the more high-tech office chairs have this level of functionality. If you tilt it too much, you will notice that your body overcompensates and your head and shoulders feel pushed forwards. A slight forward tilt of the pelvis allows the spinal curves to assume their ideal position and dissipate the weight of the body evenly through your whole structure.

2. Seat wedges are invaluable for chairs that don't have this tilt function. They are inexpensive, lightweight, and easy to carry around with you. The best place to find them is your nearest ABC™ centre because they will be designed with the correct materials, size, and angle with postural support in mind. You can, however, get some pretty good ones online. If you are travelling or find yourself without your wedge, a rolled-up towel or folded newspaper (my favourite option when travelling on planes and trains) placed under your "seat" bones can effectively raise your hips and tilt your pelvis forwards. You are aiming to have your hips higher than your knees, so that your thighs angle downwards slightly.

3. The upright back of the chair should ideally be flat because any variation of forwards or backwards tilting or contouring will either push you forwards or force you to slump.

4. Avoid chairs that are too soft or too deep because they will also force you forwards. *All* sofas cause this problem, especially if they have a deep base. Since it's comfortable to sit on, you won't likely notice its effects until you get out of it, at which point you won't breathe, move, or stand as well. The only way to minimise the damage that sofas cause is to lie on your back lengthways across them, like a bed, using only a very thin pillow to prop up your head. You could also lie on your side if you get the pillow height correct. Another alternative is to lie on the floor with a thin pillow (or use the folded towel option as taught in Chapter 7) to watch TV or read. When relaxing in the evenings, the best solution is to use a firm, L-shaped dining room chair with a seat wedge. If you must use a sofa, either lie flat or keep your time on there to a minimum and pay attention to how your body feels when you get up. Over time, you will innately recognise the damaging effects of sofa use, and it will become an easy choice to avoid it altogether.

5. There is some confusing misinformation out there that lumbar rolls help to support your spine. This is not true. All they do is apply a forwards pressure to the lower back, which may produce some relief for lower-back discomfort, but it also forces your body to slump forwards from the point where the top of the roll is placed. Your pelvis, not your lower back is supposed to support you when seated, which is why it is so important to sit on something firm and slightly angled. That way it can do its job and provide the best conditions for spinal support.

6. With car seats, have the back of the seat angled as straight as possible, and use a seat wedge to prevent your buttocks from sinking below your knees. Some car seats will allow you to take the headrest out, turn it around, and put it back in. This is a good idea to prevent the headrest from forcing your head forwards. Never remove the headrest completely, however, since it is there to prevent your head from hyperextending in the event of an accident.

7. Many people prop themselves up in bed to read, leaning against the headboard with their legs stretched out in front of them. This is a very disadvantageous position, and it will force you to slump heavily in to a forwards curve. It is better to lie flat with a very thin pillow (as taught in Chapter 7) and hold your book up to read.

8. It is nearly impossible to maintain good ergonomics and posture when you work on a laptop, especially if your put it on your legs. Your head will nearly always have to angle downwards to see the screen, so it is a good idea to use a docking station if your laptop is your primary means of working.

9. Sit at the front of your seat. Leaning back in your chair causes your weight to shift away from your ischial tuberosities (the large bony prominences at the base of your buttocks) and onto your glutes and hamstrings. These muscles are not designed to be weight-bearing surfaces, and they will end up tight and unhappy over time if you use them in this way. To make it worse, the backrest of the chair forces your spinal mechanics into a compensated state, even if you rest completely backwards. This will cause you to get stiff and sore as the day wears on. It is also very difficult to work from this position; you have to reach your arms out and round your upper back forwards to be able to reach your keyboard. Again, a silly way to sit, and one that will cause problems. The simple solution is to find the flattest, firmest chair that you can (usually the cheaper plastic or wooden ones), and sit right at the front of it with your pelvis in the neutral position. Your thighs should be angled down slightly towards your knees, with about sixty percent of the weight through your sit bones and forty percent transferred down through your heels. Your back will naturally assume a relaxed upright posture if you get this right, and as long as you get up and move around every thirty minutes or so, you will minimise the damage that sitting causes. It should look something like this:

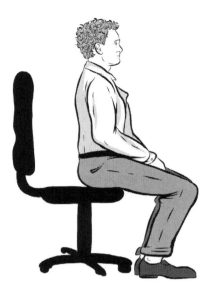

[Figure 12] Sitting on the edge of the chair encourages good posture by angling the thighs downwards.

THE ERGONOMIC CHAIR

You can get some surprisingly sophisticated "moulded" chairs these days. The problem with these chairs is that they will never allow you to sit correctly because they are specifically designed to provide you with artificial support. The basic idea is that, as you lean back on them, the curves and headrest hold you in ideal alignment. The reality, however, is that when you lean back on the chair, your muscular support system shuts off, and you're forced into a compensated position that will inevitably worsen your mechanics. These chairs are also designed in such a way that it becomes difficult, if not impossible, to sit towards the front of them; they are too soft to give pelvic support, and their shape usually doesn't accommodate a seat wedge with ease. The bottom line is that even the most expensive of ergonomic chairs will not solve the problem of sitting because your body does not need artificial support in order to work the way it was intended to work.

SWISS BALLS AND KNEELING CHAIRS

I am not a fan of either of these options, as they lead to different problems. The big, inflatable Swiss Balls may allow you to move around more consistently as you sit, but they do not provide a firm platform for your pelvis. Instead, they work in a manner similar to a sofa, causing your buttocks to sink in and your weight to be spread through your hamstrings and gluteal muscles. This type of setup makes it so that your mechanical lever system cannot naturally hold you upright, and you will need to use muscular effort (which will soon cause fatigue and leave you slumped).

Kneeling chairs can give you a more firm support, but they will tip your pelvis too far forwards leading to an overcompensation effect. This effect may, in fact, leave your lower back feeling a bit better, but it will force your head and shoulders too far forwards. Your body will have to assume an over-extended position in order to remain upright, which will also lead to fatigue and other problems over time. Additionally, knees are not designed to be mechanically loaded up for prolonged periods in the way that a kneeling chair encourages, so again, this type of chair works against your body's natural design rather than with it. Anytime you go against nature, there is an inevitable price to pay.

HOW TO OPTIMISE YOUR SITTING

Based on the information we've covered in this chapter, the best option when it comes to preserving the health of your body structure is clearly to avoid sitting. Instead, stand whenever possible. There will be times, of course, whether you are on a flight, driving to work, or enjoying dinner with your family, when this is not possible.

Whether our spines like it or not, sitting has become part of the fabric of modern life, and it is here to stay.

You probably haven't given much thought to the skill of sitting. In fact, that is a big part of the problem—most people don't even think about it, they just plop down on a chair and let gravity do its thing. There is, however, a skill to the process which is important to learn if you want to save your spine.

THE THREE GOLDEN RULES OF SITTING

When you sit, follow these three rules in order to minimise the impact that sitting has on you:

1. Sit with your pelvis in a neutral position

2. For every thirty minutes that you sit, get up and move for two to five minutes.

3. Where possible get your body corrected with ABC™ to restore your alignment and reverse the damaging effects of sitting that inevitably build up over time.

FINDING PELVIS NEUTRAL

A key point that is often misunderstood is that when your spine is relaxed, it is already in the most optimal position, allowing for the best mechanical function it can achieve given its underlying state of alignment. Knowing this is helpful when trying to put into context much of the posture and training advice that you may have received in the past. It means that forcibly changing your posture does not necessarily translate into a better or healthier body. If a particular spine has a lot of mechanical problems, its relaxed position may not look very good compared to the stereotypical perfect posture, but it does reflect its current best effort. If you try to "improve" it without realigning the primary problem bones, there will be a tradeoff of reduced function somewhere else in the body.

You will remember that the negative effect of compensation tension can easily be noticed by doing the body awareness exercise. Simply compare the quality and depth of your breath when naturally relaxed versus being in some sort of enhanced postural position that someone has told you is the correct way to sit or stand.

THE PELVIS NEUTRAL POSITION

Tilt your pelvis forwards as far as it can go, then tilt it backwards as far as it can go. The pelvis neutral position is the mid-point between these two extremes.

It is important to understand these basics, because they guide you on the best path to rebuilding your healthiest body, which is different from protecting what you currently have. Knowing the rules, however, doesn't prevent you from breaking them when doing so works in your favour—when lifting a heavy weight, for example, or assuming a sitting position. When you are under physical stress, it can be helpful to know some of the basics in terms of how to properly organise and brace your body to prevent injury. This is where learning to find the pelvis neutral position can greatly help you.

When most people stand in a typical fashion, their bum sticks out behind them. This is called an anterior pelvic tilt. The opposite is true when most people sit down; their bum tucks underneath them, and they assume a posterior pelvic tilt. Pelvis neutral is the position that exists between these two extremes. You can find it by letting your pelvis tilt forwards as far as it will go, then backwards as far as it will go, and then finding the midpoint between the two positions (you can do this when sitting or standing). When you have located this position, you should find that your transverse abdominal (TVA) muscles gently brace around your belly, almost as though a belt has tightened up. If not, you need some practice to learn how to activate them.

There are two ways to do this. One method that works well is to gently draw your belly button in towards your spine and feel your TVA tighten. Another way that works well—but is slightly different— is to imagine that you have a belt around your lower abdomen, and you are pushing your abdominals out against this belt, all the way around. While these two methods feel slightly differently from one another, they both activate your "core" to help protect your body if you're performing a heavy lift or complicated movement. If your spine is healthy, these muscles naturally kick into action and do their job. If you have had years of mechanical imbalance and postural stress, these muscles can become lazy and need to be retrained a bit in order to automatically kick in when you need them.

CORE ACTIVATION AND AWARENESS

Method 1: Position yourself in pelvis neutral and gently draw your belly button in towards your spine until you feel your core muscles tighten slightly, like a belt around your midriff.

Method 2: Imagine that you have a belt tied around your

abdomen at the level of your belly button. Independent of your breathing, try to gently brace your abdominal muscles by pushing out against this imaginary belt.

Neither method should restrict your breathing and the activation should be subtle and unstrained.

When you sit down, even if you are on a seat wedge, it is important that you find the pelvis neutral position because this places your sit bones, which are known as your ischial tuberosities, directly underneath you to support the weight of your body. If instead you sit with your bum tucked under, the weight gets pushed through your sacrum (the large central bone of your pelvis, located beneath your belt line) as well as your gluteal and hamstring muscles. Your posture will slump, and you will train imbalances into your body over time.

From this pelvis neutral position, your hip and leg muscles can optimally activate, making it much easier to stand up from a seated position. You should be able to stand up without using your arms to push on your legs. In fact, you should almost effortlessly spring up if you are sat in a decent chair, in pelvis neutral, with your TVA gently engaged. If you can't, it's a problem, and I would humbly suggest that you consider it a wake-up call with regard to the overall condition of your body. At the very least, we should each be able to handle our body weight easily and efficiently. If you cannot, the issue could be that you aren't strong enough because your activity levels have been too low to keep your legs well conditioned. Or, it could be that your chair is dipping down at the back, forcing your bum to sink in and putting you at a mechanical disadvantage. Or, it could be that your alignment is poor enough to prevent proper movement. In many cases, all three are at play, and structural correction alongside these simple lifestyle habit changes can help you regain a high level of functional fitness.

SITTING ON THE FLOOR

Sitting on the floor is arguably the most optimal of all of the sitting positions. Since your hips will twist, they'll provide a torsion force into your pelvis that can help to give a stable base from which to sit upright. Your pelvis will also directly contact the floor and take the brunt of your weight, which is what it was designed to do, unlike when you sit on a chair, where much of the weight ends up going through your hamstrings (unless you sit on the front of the chair).

If you are flexible enough to get into the normal cross-legged position without your mid-back curling forwards, you are a great candidate for floor sitting. If you can't get into the position, it means that your hips are too tight (somewhat ironically, due to too many years spent sitting). You can, instead, sit on a yoga block or a small, hard cushion. Raising your pelvis by one or two inches can make it much easier to assume the position. If you still find yourself falling forwards, use a higher block, and if that doesn't stop you from falling forwards you are probably not a great candidate for floor sitting unless you improve your mobility over time (which will occur with ABC™). You may not be able to sit for too long before your legs go to sleep, but over time, your hips will loosen, and you'll be able to maintain the position with ease.

If you have very flexible hips, the lotus position is a nice option. This classic yoga pose involves crossing your legs and placing each foot on top of the opposite thigh. There is a lot of support provided to your pelvis through passive hip external rotation, meaning that little tension is needed in your spine to stay upright. The trouble is, very few people can achieve this position.

One of the side benefits to sitting on the floor is that you must perform a full squat to get down into and up from that position. This movement is very good for your lower back and hip strength, and it is yet another way to increase your activity levels through simple changes to your daily habits. Interestingly, in the spirit of the shocking research on which this chapter is based, a study out of Brazil showed that people who cannot pass the simple test of getting up and down off the floor without support were more likely to die an early death.[44] In other words, if you improve your structural health and practice this sort of simple body weight movement regularly, you could extend your life!

WORK STANDING UP

Working while standing up is a far better option than sitting because it is an active position that involves the use of many more muscles and joints. This means that you are more maneuverable, can compensate much better for any existing mechanical problems, are far less likely to stoop, have a better-working brain, and are expending energy as you work. Sitting expends about 300 calories over an eight-hour period, whereas standing for the same timeframe burns around 1,300 calories. This type of energy expenditure whilst you are stationary has been called NEAT, or Non-Exercise Activity Thermogenesis. Standing expends a whopping 1,000 more calories per day than does sitting. Over time, that adds up and can make the difference between someone remaining at a healthy weight and becoming obese.[45] Being more active is the one of the highest-priority goals when it comes to keeping a healthy, upright body. So why not take advantage of every trick in the book (literally)! Working while standing is one of the best habits to adopt because it takes care of your posture *and* keeps you more active. It's a win, win!

It is easy to set up a standing work desk, but you must make sure that you do it correctly. You must have enough space to allow you opportunities to move around, and it must be set up at the correct height so that your monitors and keyboard are ergonomically positioned. You should take some time to work up to standing all day, since doing so will use your muscles differently than you're used to. It can take some time to adapt.

Being upright allows you to regularly shift positions, and this is important because the goal is not to stand rigidly all day long. Staying in any single position, ergonomically correct or not, can cause problems. You will naturally shift from leg to leg, you can lean against the front of the table, you can put one foot up on a footstool, or you can perch against a high stool behind you. The goal is to stay upright but also active. Again, take a break every thirty minutes and do some simple movements. This is an important part of the active and functional agenda.

STANDING WORK STATION SET-UP

Here are some ergonomic pointers for achieving a proper standing workstation set-up at home or office.

Desk: There are many stand-up brands available. You can get a fixed-height desk, which is built to a standard height, or you can get an adjustable one that moves up and down, allowing you to use it as both a standing and a sitting desk. I recommend getting an adjustable desk so that you can fine-tune it to support good posture. You can find the perfect height by standing upright in your normal, correct posture, then bend your forearms so that they are parallel to the floor. The ideal desk height is the same as the relative position of your elbow from the floor. You can tinker with the height a little bit if you want, but this is a good starting point.

Monitor: Position your monitor so that the top of your screen is aligned with your eyes. If you can angle your screen upwards slightly, it will be even easier to maintain good ergonomics as you work. Your face should be somewhere between eighteen and thirty inches away from the screen so that you don't have to move your head to see the whole screen. If you are using a laptop, you will need to get a docking station that can position your screen high enough that it meets the correct eye level. If you simply place a laptop on your standing desk, you will have to look down to see the screen, and this will cause you to stoop after a while.

Keyboard and mouse: Follow the same instructions as you did when determining your ideal desk height. Your keyboard and mouse should be directly below your hands, with your elbows resting by your sides. If you need to use the mouse often, try to position it directly in front of your body so that you don't need to twist your arm sideways in order to reach and operate it.

Shoes: We covered shoes in depth in the previous chapter, but to reiterate, it's recommended that you wear completely flat, thin and flexible-soled shoes. Going barefoot is best, or even wearing simply socks, but if you can't do this due to work restrictions, wearing shoes that keep you as close to barefoot as possible is important. Remember that a heel lift of up to one-and-a-half inches can be helpful for some people's posture.

Stool: It can be useful to have a stool to lean against if your body gets tired in the early days of switching to a stand-up work routine.

Foot Rest: Placing one of your feet up on a small foot rest can take a lot of mechanical stress out of your spine and provides a good option for you to regularly shift positions as you work.

Floor: Ideally, your floor should be concrete, wood, or another hard surface. You don't want your heels to sink into a soft rug because that will tilt your pelvis backwards and cause your posture to tilt.

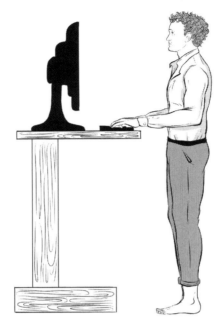

[**Figure 13**] A standing desk can make the ideal workstation.

BASIC POSTURE RULES FOR PHONES

Writing about how to properly hold a mobile phone seems almost redundant because it's obvious that your posture will fall forwards if you hold your phone on your lap whilst you use it. "Text neck" has recently become a recognised medical condition, especially among younger generations who spend a lot of time on their phones. The simple fix is to make sure that you raise your phone up to face level so that you can see the screen without bending your neck forwards. This is relatively easy to do and maintain, especially if you bring your elbow towards your chest and allow it to rest on your rib cage, taking out the need for muscular effort. I am convinced that mobile phones are causing a great deal of postural problems for people, even among patients who are getting treated in my clinic with ABC™. Nearly every day, I catch people sitting in the reception area, stooped forwards with their chin on their chest operating their phones, which are in their laps. The most effective remedy I have found for this is simply explaining that when you sit like that, your brain and spinal cord are being stretched, and your heart, lungs, diaphragm, and internal organs are all getting squashed. This reminder seems to do the trick!

BECOMING MORE ACTIVE

One of the golden rules is to get up every thirty minutes and do some movement for one or two minutes. It doesn't have to be a high-exertion activity such as a hill sprint, a simple walk around the office to get a glass of water can help a lot. A few simple movements can make a world of difference. The key is remembering to do them. Fortunately, there are several apps that you can download to help you stay committed (do a Google search on "productivity planner" or "desktop timer apps"). Even setting a repeat timer for every thirty minutes on your phone works well. Here are a few suggestions as to what you could do during your one- or two-minute break. The is not an exhaustive list, so be creative. Just get moving.

Ladder Climbs: Stand up straight, stretch one arm up as high as you can can, and bend and lift your opposite leg. Repeat with the other arm and leg as if climbing a ladder. Keep your head up and look at the tips of your fingers as you reach up.

Half Star Jumps: Keeping your head up, lift your elbows up as you jump a half step out.

Shoulder Roll: Spread your legs so they are slightly more than shoulder width apart. Slightly bend your knees and squeeze your glutes. Bend arms up to a seventy-degree angle with palms facing forwards. Rotate your shoulders backwards in a circular motion for a few repetitions, then forwards for a few repetitions.

Jog on the Spot: While looking straight ahead, do a light jog in place to get your legs and heart rate going.

Yes, No, Maybe: These are the directions in which you can gently move your neck and back. The direction is in the name. Don't force any of the movements and hold them each for ten to twenty seconds. These are not supposed to be big stretches; they are simply intended to take your joints through their normal range of motion.

NECK
For YES, bring your chin to your chest and hold, then look up at the ceiling and hold.
For NO, turn your neck to the left and hold, then to the right and hold.
For MAYBE, bring your ear to the same-side shoulder and hold. Repeat on the other side.

BACK
For YES, gently bend forward to touch your toes and hold. Don't force or bounce; you want to avoid forcing any bones forwards. Then, gently lean backwards, supporting your weight with your hands on your hips. Again, be gentle and don't force it, or you risk misaligning vulnerable bones forwards.
For NO, hold your arms out in front of you with your fingers

interlocked. Turn your trunk to the left by bringing your hands around to the side and holding. Repeat towards the other side.

For MAYBE, gently lower each arm down towards the outside of the same-side knee and hold. Repeat on the other side.

Wall Angel: Find a flat clear section of wall and stand with your back and legs pressed against it. Raise your arms above your head, keeping them straight, and place the backs of your arms and hands against the wall. Trying to keep your arms, head, back, and bum against the wall at all times, slowly lower your elbows towards your sides as far as they can go without any part of your body coming off the wall. You should feel a squeeze between your shoulder blades. Hold it for a few seconds, then shake your arm and repeat a few times. Be careful not to arch your mid back, and once again, don't force it.

Air squats, lunges, planks, and press-ups are also simple and effective exercises, but your overall options are limitless. One of my favourite solutions for long days spent in front of the computer is placing a walking treadmill under my standing desk. This allows me to slowly walk as I work. You'd be surprised how quickly you can get used to typing and walking at the same time!

THE QUICK FIX

There is one way that you can move which stands a good chance of improving your mechanics by helping to lift up vertebrae which get stuck forwards. This is a great general movement to add into your working day, on every movement break, or indeed immediately after you sit down for a period of time, or perform and exercise or movement which you think has stuck your posture forward. It is a very simple stretch-type movement, but the only thing I have discovered which allows you to improve your own alignment safely.

Here it is:

THE SELF-ADJUSTMENT MOVE

Stand up, take a deep breath in and hold it, then raise one arm straight above your head and reach up as high as you can towards the ceiling for one or two seconds. You can also raise up onto your opposite toes if you balance is good enough to allow it. Then do the opposite movement with your other arm and repeat 2-3 times both sides.

You may hear some clicks and pops in your back and even sometimes feel the bones physically realigning in the backwards direction. Afterwards you should note that you can stand straighter and breathe a little bit better. Since this is an indirect force placed onto the vertebrae, there is no guarantee that it will.

In case you are worried that anyone might think you're a bit strange for adding regular movement breaks into your days, spare a thought for what the science shows. We know that movement is crucial for brain function, and failing to move regularly is actually harmful for cognition and focus. Perhaps the modern set of office desks and chairs is why the average worker has been shown to only work for three hours per day. The rest of the hours are spent procrastinating and wasting time.

There is a lot of research showing that being more active at work can improve productivity. Facebook, for example, reported that since installing stand-up desks into their offices, employees feel more energetic throughout the day. Moving more often has also been shown to help manage work-related stress and improve levels of engagement and concentration. So if anyone says anything, just put on your propeller hat on and teach them some science.

BRYONY'S UNWINDING STORY

Entrepreneur, 21

I first started receiving ABC™ after seeing chiropractors since I was ten years old. It was the generic type, and I went just to keep a healthy spine. I stopped that at age eighteen because I didn't feel it was benefiting me anymore. At the time, I was doing a lot of ballet and started experiencing lower back pains and pain in my knees from all of the exercise and the stretching I was doing. I felt it was time to see a new chiropractor, and I ended up at SpineCentral (Richard's Clinic in London). I quickly realised that they practice a very different type of chiropractic care, which worked much better for me.

I found that my back not only became pain free, it also become a lot more flexible. I was able to take my foot from behind my back and pull it over my head, which is not something most people are aspiring to but it was very useful for me as a ballerina, and that was the first time I've ever been able to do that! The other great change is that I've noticed I no longer get a stiff neck after sitting and working at my computer all day. I like to feel nice and upright, and ABC™ has helped me to maintain a really good posture even with all of the work I do running an online business.

CHAPTER 9

Moving Well

"First move well, then move often"

—Gray Cook

T his book is about the importance of alignment, why it goes wrong, how to regain it, and how to maintain it. But, just like a car, the reason that you fix its mechanical problems is so that you can drive it, enjoy the ride, and go to interesting places.

Consider your body to be the vehicle you use to travel through life. The funny thing is that human beings have a remarkable ability to live for surprisingly long periods of time in a neglected vehicle— one that is sedentary, poorly aligned, and generally unhealthy. One can go for fifty or sixty years on a diet of fast food burgers, crisps, and fizzy drinks with zero exercise without appearing to break down too badly (of course, you would be fairly miserable as a result of this lifestyle, even though you'd eventually think it was a normal way to feel). Yet, sooner or later, the game is up, and we are all held accountable for our past choices. Looking after your body so that it goes the distance should be an obvious goal, but a long life alone is the wrong outcome to focus on; it entirely misses the point of healthy living. Longevity is a hopeful offshoot of living true to the laws of nature. The real benefit of being healthy is that you get to do more, experience more, and enjoy your life more every day that you're above ground. As the old saying goes, life is about the journey, not the destination.

The best reason to restore your alignment is to enable you to move correctly, enjoy your body, and do incredible things with it along the way. As a fair-exchange bonus, you also get greater health benefits from any movement that you do. A well-aligned skeleton moves freely in all directions, affording you the privilege of effortless movement, greater stimulation of your brain, better repair and remodeling of your joints, freedom to fully breathe, optimally pump blood, and go about life pain-free with a greatly reduced risk of injury. When good alignment comes together with sufficient movement, one arguably has the most powerful positive momentum builder for his health.

When you go for a long walk, run, or great gym session, you release built-up stress. What is the first thing that you want to do when you get home from that exercise session? Eat a healthy meal, of course. When you do that, you sleep well. You then wake up from a great night's sleep, your mind is sharp, and you feel powerful at work. Your energy stays steady and abundant, so you feel inspired to take regular breaks and feed your body further nutritious movement. Then, what do you want to do at the end of the day? You want to work out again. As you can see, the cycle is likely to repeat. When you live this way, it becomes clear that movement is one of the most important keys to a healthy body and mind as well as a productive, effective life.

Good alignment is a key ingredient because, without it, movement and exercise likely will, at least eventually, become self-defeating. Who wants to work out if their back just stiffens up or they are gasping for breath due to limited chest function? Equally, what motivation or possibility is there to move if you have sciatica? Even if you do find the will power to push through your poor alignment, an injury will eventually risk derailing your progress and deflating your ambitions to continue. I've seen well-intentioned, hard-working, ambitious people fall victim to this pattern all too often, and it's a shame. One's efforts in the areas of movement and exercise can and should be enjoyable and self-reinforcing. In order to reach that lofty goal, you must first focus on restoring healthy alignment. If you don't, sooner or later you'll be sidelined, out of the race, and back at the mechanic's, up on the blocks.

NOT ALL MOVEMENT IS CREATED EQUAL

You may be one of the few people who have gone through life without paying attention to your alignment or movement and haven't suffered any ill effects. You could, therefore, be tempted to dismiss my message that alignment matters. But, before you do, consider the reality that your body works on a functional spectrum. Only once it has accumulated enough mechanical dysfunction will it no longer be able to compensate for problems. It is at this point that pain, injury, and other ill consequences will begin.

Consider that each of your body parts comes primed for a certain number of uses throughout its lifetime. In fact, genetically speaking, science has revealed that if we could perfect our lifestyles, we would be able to sustain healthy life for about 120 years. Of course, most of us are living lifestyles that are not exactly picture-perfect, and so we can't expect to reach such advanced ages, at least not as things stand. Medical breakthroughs may change that in the future, but for now, our best bet for longevity comes from mastering lifestyle, and movement is one of the key spokes on the wheel of wellness.

A simple way to understand the impact of movement is to consider that if you correctly move a well-aligned joint though its full range of motion, you will only use up one duty cycle. If that same movement is executed poorly with incorrect alignment of the joint surfaces, you may use up several duty cycles. Obviously, the faster you use up your duty cycles, the sooner that joint will degenerate and "wear out."

Let's put that into perspective. If you were to walk 10,000 steps per day, which is the accepted recommendation for healthy, active people, that would lead to 70,000 steps in a week, which would total 3.5 million steps in a year, and approximately thirty-five million steps over ten years. Now imagine if, over the next ten years, you took each of your millions of steps with your body stuck forwards and twisted, with one foot rolled in, the other one turned out, one hip higher than the other, and the opposite shoulder lower and rolled forwards. You can imagine, I'm sure, that there is a significant increased usage of duty cycles compared to a person who took their thirty-five million steps whilst in good alignment. Of course, we don't just walk; we also run, lift weights, clean the house, play sports, and perform myriad other movements throughout a typical day. Each of these movements comes with a higher tax on the body if alignment and posture are poor. We are designed to handle a high number of duty cycles over a long period of time, going the distance and staying fit and agile into old age. On the other hand, we are *not* designed to handle a large number of exaggerated and taxed duty cycles because of poor alignment.

I have seen rugby players in my clinic as young as twenty-six years old whose neck X-rays look like they could be those of someone thirty to forty years older. Quite simply, they have used up their duty cycles far too early because poor alignment created by the trauma of their sport met with a high intensity of movement and wore out the joints before their time. Granted, that's a fairly extreme example of a person stressing their structure, but it is hardly uncommon. Millions of people around the world participate in high-impact contact sports such as rugby and football, which are likely to leave them suffering later in life. There is no reason why these sports cannot be enjoyed. The issue is simply that they don't come without consequence, and participating in them will create a greater need for care and attention to be placed on maintaining good alignment and mechanics.

A much more common scenario that I see on an almost daily basis is the person who "just bent down to pick up a pen," and their lower back "just went out." A disc has herniated, and they are left keeled over in agony, unable to move, with a significant injury. People are often quite surprised when this happens to them and feel somewhat hard done by. How could such an innocent movement wreak such havoc? The truth is that they have been bending, moving, and performing their sitting, sleeping, and standing habits incorrectly for years, burning through their duty cycles. They managed to get away with it for a while, until the inevitable time when they no longer could. Think of yourself as a million-pound supercar. You can still go fast with your wheels out of alignment and the handbrake on. It's impressive and enjoyable for a while, but sooner or later, you won't be going anywhere.

This does not mean that exercise should be feared or that there is necessarily a big trade-off between being fit now and being riddled with arthritis when you are older. There is, however, a balance that needs to be met. If you are active in pursuing good alignment with the use of structural correction and the other lifestyle advice in this book, you can do more in the way of exercise without falling foul of your biological tolerance. Lots of movement in good alignment is the goal.

It is worth remembering that exercise, as we have come to know it, is not really the same thing as movement. From the dawn of humankind to around 10,000 BC, hunter-gatherers were on-the-go, continuously running, balancing, hunting, foraging, jumping, crawling, building, manipulating tools, carrying, throwing, and fighting—all literally in the name of survival. A day in the life of a typical hunter-gatherer was highly calorific and stimulating for their body structure. It was during these times as hunter-gatherers that our genes evolved, and over the past 10,000 years they have changed very little. In fact, the modern-day human genome is thought to be less than 0.02% different from that of our hunter-gatherer ancestors. This means that movement is hard-wired into our genes, and as a result, it is still an expected and required biological stimulus in order to express optimal health.

The best way to think about movement is as an essential nutrient just like vitamin D or Omega-3 fats. Your body needs movement in order to sustain healthy function. The physiological benefits of movement are so nutritious, in fact, that if you could bottle up its health benefits and put them into a pill, it would be the greatest-selling drug of all time. The research around the benefits of movement is truly astonishing. Several volumes could be written on that subject alone. Exercise has been shown to reduce the incidence of cancer, stroke, heart disease, osteoporosis, depression, anxiety, gallstones, pain, osteoporosis, obesity, and diabetes. Frankly, you name the ailment, and exercise has likely cured it for someone. The really interesting result of many of the completed studies is that participants weren't asked to run a marathon every week. More often than not, the exercise intervention was as simple as taking a fifteen-minute walk in one direction, and then turning around and walking back. As few as thirty minutes of walking per day can have quite profound health implications—not because exercise is a great treatment strategy, but because movement, as an essential nutrient, is required for the normal healthy expression of your physiology.

The key point to grasp is that if you can figure out how to get more active during your normal days, you can take care of something really important in your health. Getting in 10,000 steps per day is pretty easy if you walk to work or park the car a fifteen-minute walk from work. Walk to the shops, take up dancing, take the stairs, use a stand-up desk, employ forced movement breaks every twenty minutes, and implement walking meetings. There are many ways that you can get more active during a normal day without exhausting yourself or burdening your routine. Exercise can absolutely become a part of your strategy to fulfill your movement requirements, but the place to start making changes is by addressing your sedentary habits and deliberately enhancing your movement patterns throughout a typical day.

It's fascinating to think that exercise is very much a modern-day invention, becoming a "thing" during the 1970s with the advent of aerobics. The new approaches to getting fit do come with some downsides, not least of which is the temptation to do too much in too short a period of time. Cramming a full-body weights session into thirty minutes at lunchtime is not only fairly stressful but it may also train imbalances into your body if done incorrectly. Modern-day work schedules make it difficult to stay active, but being sedentary all week only to become a fitness warrior on the weekend may be self-defeating strategy for a body that is already overworked and under-recovered.

Studies have shown that brief bouts of exercise, even if they are intense, are not sufficient to overcome the damaging health effects of an overall sedentary work and home life. This doesn't even take into account the negative impact that exercise, when done poorly, can have on your alignment and mechanics. By its very nature, exercise is a double-edged sword with the potential both to build you up and break you down. If done well, exercise and sports can be incredibly healthy and rewarding attributes of your lifestyle. Personally, I have gotten more joy out of competitive sports than I have from just about anything else in life, so I am certainly not recommending that you avoid these activities. Rather, I am stressing the importance of doing them well and being aware of the impact they can have upon your alignment because that is the key factor in determining the longevity, robustness, and health of your body. Above and beyond that, I am stressing the importance of increasing the amount that you move your body every day as well as the quality of the movement that you undertake. This can include exercise, but it must go beyond that to become a generally active and physical lifestyle. That's the real key to success with physical health: move often and move well with a foundation of good alignment. If you exercise already or are keen to begin, protecting your alignment and avoiding unnecessary physical stress should be an ever-present guiding principle by which you train.

KEY MISTAKES TO AVOID WHEN EXERCISING

Remember that not all movements are created equal. It is perfectly possible to take an exercise that is good for you, perform it poorly, and have it create more harm than good.

THE STRAIGHT TRUTH

The number one rule when working out is to pay attention to any forces that could misalign your back bones forwards. Generally, this happens if there is forceful flexion (forwards) or extension (backwards) movement put through your spine.

Performing a heavy lift or pull with poor posture can leave you stuck forwards, as can pretty much any exercise or movement done with poor form. It is critical to be self-aware and think about your posture as you work out or play sports. Any time you are excessively or forcefully bending forwards or extending backwards, you risk creating forwards-stuck back bones. The risk goes up if your technique is lazy or flawed. Being present and deliberate with your movement can prevent a lot of the mechanical problems associated with exercise.

Certain movements such as sit ups are almost certain to cause mechanical problems, and ironically, they are not even a good exercise. Sit-ups are also now considered by most spine health experts as harmful for the lower back, but the mechanism behind why they cause harm was poorly understood until recently (they lever the vulnerable bones forward). Your abdominal core musculature can be trained in far more effective ways without placing mechanical strain on your body. The plank exercise, for example, is perfectly suited to this task.

You can also forcibly push a bone forwards by putting a heavy barbell on your back and doing deep heavy back squats. It is not uncommon for athletes to feel light-headed during a movement like this. The commonly held belief is that, under the strain, there is a drop in blood flow to the brain, resulting in that floaty feeling. That is only part of the story, however. When you consider the mechanics of the body, a more likely explanation for the dizziness is that, under the weight of the barbell, a vertebrae got forcibly misaligned forwards, lost its leverage, and is now putting an adverse mechanical tension on the spinal cord and brain stem with neurological consequences.

The same mechanism is in play when you feel light-headed after getting up quickly from a sofa or out of the car. The chair was previously not supporting your lower back, it got stuck forwards, and now you have neurological tension. Low blood pressure can lead to the same symptoms, but this mechanism should also be appreciated since it is real-time feedback from your body with regard to the impact of your physical choices.

Along similar lines, have you ever got up from a sports massage and felt light-headed and dreamy, like you were ready to fall asleep?

This is not just relaxation. This is mechanical pressure on your spinal cord caused from the massage, which released the compensatory muscle tension and also probably pushed forwards any vulnerable back bones—again, with neurological consequences.

On the other end of the scale, we have extreme backward bending movements, like the yoga bridge or the classic extension over a large inflatable gym ball. These two commonly used exercises can force spinal segments forwards quite easily because of the strong cantilever effect of your body's mass moving backwards. As Newton so cleverly figured out, for every action, there is an equal and opposite reaction, which means that as you bend back, something must be pushed forwards to compensate. Great care should be taken if you ever do these movements. Better still, they should be avoided altogether by most people.

The advice is not to avoid forward flexion or backwards extension completely, but rather to avoid careless and unfocused use of these movements where a large force is "pushed" through a section of your spine. Another example is doing heavy bicep curls with your upper back and neck bent forwards, pulling your mid-back bones forwards with every repetition. There are literally thousands of ways that you can exercise poorly and create these uncontrolled forwards forces on your body, which is why the knowledge you have gained on biomechanics by reading this far is so important. Once you understand how anything works, that knowledge and the end result are both more useful to you. Who wouldn't want their own body to be more useful and to experience fewer problems?

A simple way to know if your workout routine or sport is causing your mechanical mischief is to take note of how you feel after a workout. Feeling tired is quite normal, but feeling tight or locked up in your back or neck is not a good sign. If your spinal range of motion is more restricted than when you started, some part of your training has aggravated your condition or created new problems for you.

With this level of awareness, you can assess every movement you do and determine if it helped or hindered.

In the past, I've been criticised by personal trainers (and others) for highlighting the importance of taking care not to inadvertently push spinal bones forwards during exercise. The standard response is, "You are designed to bend forwards and backwards; it's part of normal healthy movements, and if you don't train in flexion, how can you expect to ever get strong in flexion?" These points are all true, to a certain degree. A balanced, well-aligned and functionally fit spine will handle flexion or extension without getting misaligned. The key point is that there are few people in this day and age who fit that criteria. Nearly everyone is working a desk job where they sit for eight to ten hours per day, has experienced a car crash or two, commutes to and from work, sits down in the evening, and has had multiple accidents, falls, and injuries throughout their life. When you take into account the impact of poor movement patterns in sport; the use of unhealthy shoes; and the ways in which pillows, mattress, and sofas have distorted one's skeletal frame, you can see how the average modern-day human commonly has major mechanical problems. Some of these problems will be quite progressed since they are likely to have been there for a decade or longer. These problematic injuries can be unstable and easy to aggravate. Just as if you were to keep prodding a sore patch of skin, it can never truly heal. You certainly do not want to be aggravating old injuries or creating new stuck-forwards sections of your spine. A heavy workout may leave you feeling tired, but it should never leave you feeling locked up and less flexible or imbalanced in your body.

As is the case with my sitting, sleeping, and standing recommendations, the importance of following this advice increases if you are receiving structural correction. Once meningeal adhesions are released and your body starts to unwind and loosen, it becomes easier for a period of time to upset the mechanical balance of your body because it is no longer wound up in a protective tightness. While it may appear a nuisance, or that you are somehow more fragile than you used to be, the truth is that this is a good thing. You are not more fragile; rather, you are less able to get away with bad habits without noticing the impact on your mechanical function. Your body is a precision instrument, and it needs to be cared for as such. You can't take a Ferrari off-road and have it come back looking and driving the same. That doesn't mean that a Ferrari is inherently flawed; it means that you need to respect the way it is designed to work. Thankfully, a human skeleton has the ability to compensate for problems and paint over much of the rust that forms over time. This helps you to keep going despite the fact that you have accumulated injuries. But remember, those injuries come at the cost of reduced function, and restoring function comes with the added requirement of needing to learn healthy movement patterns and lifestyle habits to support it. This is a fair tradeoff and one that I would personally choose any day of the week.

The good news is that one of the great benefits of going through structural correction with ABC™ is that you will naturally assume an ideal alignment when playing your chosen sport or doing your favourite exercises. I frequently hear patients report with surprise how much farther they can hit the golf ball, how much heavier weight they can lift, how much faster they can serve the tennis ball, how much better they can run, how much more balanced or strong they are when skiing, and how they recover much faster afterwards, all without having trained or practiced any harder or differently. When your alignment is correct, your athleticism, performance, and recovery is optimised, but you do still need to be aware of how you perform so that you don't create new problems.

Once you have learned how to move without upsetting your mechanics, you have a foundation upon which you can build as high as you like, achieving the level of fitness you desire without the burden of injury. The fundamental fact that we cannot escape is that many sports are going to be troublesome for your alignment. They involve fast, explosive, and often, unpredictable movements. You may fall, be tackled, have to lift something heavy, accelerate quickly, stop suddenly or find that your form becomes lazy when you are tired. It is almost inevitable that mechanical problems will be created though sport. The more active you are, the greater your need for true structural correction care.

CORE CONTROL

Nearly everyone who comes to my practice has heard of core strength and its importance. You may find it interesting that core strength is a concept that was simply created one day and marketed into popularity. The idea of core strength being important came off the back of a couple of research papers in the 1990s that showed that patients with lower back pain had a small delay in the timing of their abdominal muscle contractions. From that revelation sprang up an entire industry. This has created a lot of misconceptions about what core muscles are and how they should work. The prevailing belief is that you need to keep your core muscles strong so that your back can be stable. The hypothesis that instability is the cause of back pain has led many people to try to continuously tighten their abdominals and tuck their pelvises under. The reality is that the core muscles do not work independently of the rest of the body, and the lower back does not become unstable if your abdominals become weak. This means that there is no need to be continuously bracing your abs or relentlessly training then. Developing core awareness is, however, quite important because the abdominal muscles (such as the transverse abdominis) play an important role in stabilising your body when you put it through demanding movements.

If your alignment is off and years of sedentary living have altered your movement patterns, it is certainly possible to perform exercises with no core awareness, which can leave you vulnerable to further injury. The classic example is someone performing a press-up with their spine and abdomen drooping towards the floor. This is poor form, and the forces placed onto the spine during a lazy press-up can easily force your lower and mid back bones forwards. The simple fix is to activate your core to prevent this drooping while keeping your posture strong and controlled throughout the movement. The same goes for any heavy lifting, pushing, or pulling movements. Learning how to properly activate your core is key to exercising safely and moving correctly (the two best ways to do this were covered in Chapter 8). Whilst you could choose to strengthen your core with various exercises like plank pose, you do not need to walk around with your core muscles perpetually engaged in order to prevent injury. Think in terms of your body working as one complete system with no single part being any more important that another. This appreciation, together with the relentless pursuit of proper form and skilful movements, will help you progress with your training and stay injury-free.

SCAPULA CONTROL

Your scapula are the triangular shoulder blade bones on either side of your back. They play a valuable role as the mobile platform to which various muscles attach to keep your shoulder joints strong and stable. Just as with your core musculature, it is possible to be lazy in the way you control your shoulders during exercise. Failing to properly activate and stabilise your scapulas by retracting them downwards and inwards can leave the shoulder joints vulnerable to injury during complex or strenuous movements. You can also easily place unnatural forces on your spine that could cause forwards misalignments. It is worth doing some online research or asking your chiropractor or personal trainer to teach you how to correctly retract or engage your shoulders during exercise. It is a skill that is hard to describe, but once you have it, you don't forget it, and it will become an easy and natural part of your training. You can engage your scapula with your arm in any position. Try this simple exercise:

ENGAGING SHOULDER STABILISERS

Stand up straight with your arms by your sides. Visualise your shoulder blade, and then try to pull it down and closer in towards your back without moving your shoulder or arm. This is possible because of a muscle called serratus anterior, which exists solely for this purpose. When you get it right, it feels like a tightness or an internal pressure beneath your shoulder blade. Your shoulder will feeler tighter and more secure.

FLAWLESS TECHNIQUE

Not all movement is created equal. It's perfectly possible to move in ways that create all manner of mechanical problems for yourself. Spend a hilarious few minutes on YouTube watching "funny gym fails" videos, and you will quickly learn that people do silly things in the gym. Even a good athlete with great body awareness who outwardly appears muscular and fit can be inadvertently stressing his alignment and developing an imbalance through errors in his technique.

My personal philosophy is that if you don't do it properly, don't do it at all. It's simply not worth it. The heavier the weight or greater the number of repetitions you do, the more important it is to flawlessly execute the movement. Every movement has a correct technique, one that respects your joint mechanics. Squatting, lunging, bench pressing, deadlifting, pull-ups, press-ups, planks, running, tennis, swimming, rowing—they all have many technique pointers to learn before they can be done properly. Even walking, believe it or not, can be done poorly enough to create problems over time.

Never assume that you have the correct technique without having deliberately learned or been taught by someone who knows their stuff. Thankfully, getting this instruction is easier than ever with resources like Google and Youtube. For people who enjoy lifting weights, I highly recommend the book *How To Become A Supple Leopard* by Dr. Kelly Starrett. He expertly breaks down the key parts of each movement so that you can perform it flawlessly. It never fails to surprise me how even the simplest of movements can have a multitude of small steps to master before it can be perfectly executed.

START WITH THE BASICS

Before you move onto more advanced exercises or sports techniques, ensure that you have mastered the basic movements and strength patterns. I've learned this lesson the hard way. Take, for example, the humble press-up. This move is pretty easy for most physically fit people. Yet, if you force yourself to do the full movement slowly with perfect form, not allowing for any shortcuts or cheats, it suddenly becomes ten times harder. This is humbling, but a good lesson indeed because unless you have earned the right to progress, you risk injury by attempting more difficult moves. In the long run, you will get much farther through consistent training than from intense periods of training followed by forced periods of down time to recover from injuries. Build slowly and methodically in your chosen sport or exercise. Always be aware that we have an incredible capacity to "cheat" by lazily performing movements or performing them in an altered way that makes them seem easier. Ultimately, that choice leaves you imbalanced and injury prone.

AVOID GETTING STUCK IN A RUT

The human machine is incredibly efficient at adapting to whatever position, posture, or movement you most frequently engage in. Your brain and body are always learning and evolving. In order to prevent injuries, protect your alignment, and keep progressing with your fitness, you must regularly change up your training routine. If we return to the example of the push-up, there are many variations even for this one simple movement. You can do wide drop, narrow drop, pseudo plank (where you lean forwards), torpedo push-ups, tricep push-ups, decline push-up, explosive clapping push-ups, battle ram push-ups, one arm push-ups, and on and on! Varying the technique or style by changing the intensity, repetitions, weight, and/or body position can keep you from overtraining using a particular movement and will ensure that your body continues to adapt and improve. If you are always doing the same routine, you risk training an imbalance into your body. You will also get less back from your body in return.

IF YOU ARE SERIOUS ABOUT PROGRESS, HIRE A COACH

Most people I have met through my practice are busy professionals who want their pursuit of health to serve them, not take over their life. Many of us just don't have the time to learn about exercise science or put together a well-balanced training program. The simple fix is to invest in someone who does. By paying a coach, not only will you be accountable to show up and do the work but you will also have someone on your team who can ensure that you do the right training, learn the correct technique, and make real progress. Trying to figure out elite-level fitness on your own is quite challenging, which is why I am a huge fan of investing in a trainer or coach to make your life easier and a solid foundation of fitness inevitable.

BE CAUTIOUS OF STRETCHING AND FOAM ROLLING

One of the first thing new patients often ask me is, "Are there any stretches I can do to help?" My response is usually, "Yes, there are many stretches you can do, but they don't solve the problem." By this stage in your reading, you know that tight muscles are performing the job of stabilising your structure, which is why stretching them out is usually not a good idea. At best, doing so provides only temporary relief, and at worst, it destabilises your mechanics and may lead to worse pain. Stretching simply doesn't address the primary cause of the problem.

The research is also very clear on the fact that stretching before exercise actually *increases* your chances of injury. This should be of no surprise because the body doesn't compensate as well for its problems when you stretch it out. If you then subject it to the rigours of sport, something is more likely to give out on you.

That doesn't mean you shouldn't warm up. It simply means that stretching is not a good warm up. It is far more effective to do gentle functional body weight movements to get your body ready for sport. If stretching is of limited benefit, however, why do so many people want to do it? The answer, I believe, is that stretching just feels good. There's a sense of relief that comes from a deep hamstring stretch, for example. If you enjoy it, feel free to stretch, but remember to respect your body mechanics and don't force the movement. Pay attention to how stable your posture is afterwards by breathing in and out and letting your body slump and relax. If you are folding forwards more than you were before, you have mechanically worsened your body by stretching, and you need to either adapt what you are doing or stop stretching.

The effect of foam rolling is not much different and can cause a lot of mechanical problems, especially if you roll your back over a roller. I have had several patients over the years who plateaued early in their care and had the same pain continue to return a few days after correction. Upon lengthy and usually frustrating enquiry, it eventually became clear that they had been told by some outside authority to roll backwards over the foam roller to stretch out their spine. This activity is guaranteed to worsen one's alignment because the pressure placed on the spine directly forces bones forwards into positions from which they cannot be retrieved. The result? You feel nice and loose immediately after rolling, but feel pain later on as your body has to compensate for the problems that have been caused. Mobility is a key part of structural health, but not when it comes at the expense of good alignment and mechanics.

Before I learned about structural correction and why bodies go wrong, I used to stretch all the time, and the frustrating thing was that I frequently injured my calf muscles when running. These days, that does not happen. I don't stretch, and my calves are robust, even when I run long distances in minimal barefoot-style trainers. Another interesting ABC™ related experience is that, after an adjustment, you will often notice that your flexibility is dramatically improved. How could this be if no muscles were stretched out in the process of correction? The answer is that with correct alignment, your body can let go of the compensation tightness because it is no longer needed. You become more flexible and mobile without stretching.

A WORD ON YOGA, PILATES, AND SIMILAR PRACTICES

Some of the most challenging patients I've helped had, over the years, have been yoga instructors. It can be an uphill struggle to get their structure balanced because the next time they go into a deep, forwards bend, shoulder stand, or backwards bend, they again pull or push something forwards, making it difficult for their body to stabilise and unwind. I realise that this may sound somewhat questionable since many people believe that yoga is the gold standard for restoring posture and mobility. Not so. Yoga and Pilates can be very helpful for loosening and strengthening a dysfunctional body, but they can never truly correct bone alignment. If a vertebrae is stuck forwards, it is not possible to move or activate your muscles in any way that can bring it back. You can become looser, you can become stronger, and you can gain better mind-body awareness and control through these disciplines, but you can't quite get to the root cause of the problem. At their best, they are helpful activities for overall fitness and stress reduction. They can serve as a fantastic guide for healthy living and deep personal growth. Many people find that they feel much better if they do these practices, which is a great. But, at their worst—especially if your spine is particularly problematic or your technique is flawed—you can cause yourself bigger problems by worsening your alignment. It is worth remembering that yoga, and to a lesser degree Pilates (which tends to focus more on core exercises than mobility), is a balanced sport for balanced bodies. If you choose to go down either of these paths, listen carefully to your body, and never push beyond your limits.

DON'T DO TOO MUCH IN ONE GO

Many amateur athletes (and even professional athletes) train too hard and for too long at one time. It is important to protect your alignment, but it is equally important to safeguard your health. Raising your heart rate and effort level to the point of being breathless and maintaining that for long periods of time is quite stressful to the body. This is why, every year, you hear about marathon runners who suddenly died during a race. They were apparently fit and healthy, yet their heart just gave up on them. It's a tough concept to wrap your head around. The reason these tragedies happen is that these athletes were chronically under-recovered and over-trained. Whilst they had trained to run hard and fast for a long time, they hadn't conditioned their aerobic metabolism to be able to safely handle the workload.

The solution is to make sure you correctly and safely build your fitness. True aerobic training is extremely safe and health enhancing because it builds your fitness, improves your metabolism, stabilises your body chemistry, and trains you to burn fat, all without unduly stressing your body. I have found that true aerobic training soon becomes positively addictive. It is as though your body starts craving low-intensity movement.

You can train your aerobic system with many different types of exercise. The simple rule is to always maintain your heart rate in the aerobic zone, which is worked out with the following formula:

$$180 - (your\ age) = Your\ Aerobic\ Heart\ Rate$$
$$e.g\ 180 - 36 = 144$$

If you are looking to safely increase your level of movement and improve your fitness over time, this is arguably the wisest way to do it. You can train aerobically by walking fast, jogging, running, cycling, rowing, dancing, swimming, body weight training, and many other activities. Slowly build your heart rate to your aerobic zone, which, in the example above, is 144 beats per minute. Maintain that heart rate for as long as you wish to train, and then spend ten minutes slowing down or walking to cool down correctly. When you first begin this type of training you may notice that just a fast walk takes you to the limit of your aerobic zone. Even if it feels easy, don't be tempted to go beyond it, even by one or two beats per minute. Maintain your aerobic heart rate, and as the sessions and weeks roll by you will find that you are able to train more and more intensely while maintaining your aerobic zone. Eventually, you'll be running, swimming, or cycling as fast as you were previously, but without the undue stress on your physiology. This is the healthy way to get fit. Of course, you will need to purchase a chest strap heart rate monitor in order to do this type of training. There are many cost-effective options available and a quick online search will let you know your options. Go for one that straps to your chest, because these are much more accurate than the ones that measure through a sensor on your wrist.

DELAYED ONSET MUSCLE SORENESS

There will inevitably be times when you overdo it with regard to exercise and get the dreaded DOMS (Delayed Onset Muscle Soreness). You'll have an amazing workout and wake up the next day to find yourself sore from head to toe and cursing your previous day's good intentions. This is just the start of your discomfort, however, because Day Two is usually worse, and the pains can linger for three or four days if you did a *really* good job. If you ask any athlete, they'll all have suggestions for reducing or preventing DOMS. The frustrating thing is that, according to current exercise science, there is no known cure for DOMS. The micro tears, swelling, and healing response are simply a painful passage you must endure in the pursuit of your training goals.

At last, that's what I *thought*—until I showed up for my ABC™ session four years ago with such bad DOMS that I couldn't raise my arms above my head. I had, as usual, gone overboard at CrossFit two days before. It could have been the one hundred pull ups or the fifty squat thrusts (just ask any CrossFitter; it's a great way to train—if you want to be forever sore and eventually have an injury take you down). I was suffering and miserable. My chiropractor took me through the ABC™ protocol, and ten minutes later said, "Try raising your hands above your head now." To my amazement, I could do so effortlessly, without any pain or tightness. My muscles were still a bit sore if I poked them, but I could move around freely without squeaking or moaning. To this day, ABC™ is the only significant treatment or relief that I have found for DOMS, and I've tried many. It doesn't instantly fix the micro tears in your muscles, but by taking the twist out of your structure, it removes the adverse mechanical tension from your skeleton and allows it to relax. When the tensions are gone, the pain is gone. You will likely have to experience this for yourself to believe it. Ever since that moment, if I over-train or otherwise become sore, the first thing I do is get adjusted so that I can stop my moaning. Miraculous!

IS THERE AN EXERCISE THAT WILL FIX MY BACK?

There are loads of exercises you can do to strengthen your body and improve your postural fitness. This is not, however, the same as correcting your structure. There is no such thing as true corrective exercise, but that does not take anything away from the importance of doing it. My intention with this book was never to bombard you with specific exercises. First of all, many books have been written that present those; you can easily pick one up online right this moment if you wish. When you undergo true structural correction, these exercises become a choice to improve your health and athleticism rather than a requirement to stay pain-free or rebuild your posture. When you address the root cause of the problem, your body will hold itself up perfectly and effortlessly without any muscular effort required. Over time, the remodeling and rehabilitative process that occurs through your entire neuromuscular skeletal system results in a robust and well-functioning body.

The simplest way to put it is that restoring alignment will give you your body back, daily movement will strengthen it, and together, they will transform your health.

RICARDO'S UNWINDING STORY

Personal Trainer and Music Teacher, 26

Two years ago, my health was in a bad way, and I couldn't live my life. I was having intense daily migraines and was pretty much bedridden and very worried about my future. My livelihood as a personal trainer depended upon me being able to be physically active and I didn't know which way to turn. I'd been to see my GP and various specialists, and no one could figure out why I had the headaches. Within a few minutes of meeting Richard, he had located what he believed to the cause, which was surprising, and I've got to say, it made me somewhat skeptical, given my past experiences.

True to his word, however, when I started the sessions my headaches almost immediately resolved, and I also noticed my posture improved as did my mood and my sleep, surprisingly. That's been one of the biggest things that I've noticed, because when your sleep improves so does your stress, your mood, and your relationships. I noticed that I also got stronger in the gym, able to lift heavier weight and perform more difficult body weight movements with better balance and ease. It's hard to describe just how much better you feel. You get rid of all the little niggles you've had for years, the neck pain, the back pain, the shoulder problems, all the common issues that you experience daily all go away, and you are able to live your life more fully. You want to do more, move more, and do things that you have been putting off because too much headspace has been taken up by pain, tiredness, and loss of trust in your body.

CHAPTER 10

Moving Forward

"Good health is a crown on the head of a well person that only a sick person can see."

—*Robin Sharma*

t was March 2010, and I was coming to the end of a glorious four months in Cape Town, South Africa. I'd spent as much time as I could kitesurfing in the ice-cold waves of the Atlantic Ocean. The conditions there are some of the best in the world for this sport, and the backdrop of Table Mountain provides jaw-dropping natural beauty that makes it a very special place to be.

Most days, I found myself in a blissful state, mixing up all of the dynamic elements of doing something challenging that I loved with intense focus and repetitive practice, free from distractions, in the perfect environment. All of that came together to create an amazing sense of flow. If you've ever been really into sport or have a vocation you love or a hobby that you get lost in, you appreciate the state of flow of which I speak as the ultimate state to be in. Perhaps it was this heightened sense, or maybe it was just coincidence, but on my final afternoon on the water, I saw something that left an indelible imprint on my mind. As I surfed in and out of the waves, practicing my transitions and jumps and loving every second of it, I glanced up to see a real master at work in front of me. He was absolutely flawless and mesmerising to watch as he masterfully surfed the 5m swell. I assumed that he was a professional, because Cape Town is somewhat of a mecca for kitesurfing talent (myself not included). It was one of the most enjoyable times I've ever had on the water, weaving in and out of the waves, following the master, mimicking his moves and feeling in-the-flow.

I finished up my session, and as I was folding away my kite, I glanced up again to see this same surfer charge at full speed towards the beach and lift his kite to launch himself into a vertical jump, which also acted like a break. As he rose up, he kicked off his board, caught it in his hand, smoothly floated down onto the sand, and jogged up the beach with his kite stalled above his head. He motioned for someone to help land his kite, and since I was there, I jumped up and helped him out. He jogged up the beach to say Thank You, and that is when I got one of the greatest lessons of my life. Not only was this French man an amateur rider, he was a vividly healthy man in his mid 70s. I was blown away when he told me his age. To recognise that it is possible to maintain such great athleticism, fitness, and function well into your 70s is truly inspiring. Above and beyond that, I realised the gift that peak physical health gives you: the ability to continue doing and mastering that which you love in life, unrestricted by physical, mental, or energetic drains. At that moment, I set the intention to be kitesurfing and performing handstands into my 80s, and hopefully beyond!

My snowboarding accident unfortunately set me back temporarily, but in the end, it has proven to be the greatest blessing in my quest to reach this goal. It led me to ABC™, which healed my body and unlocked levels of athleticism and health I never thought possible. Introducing it into my practice has reinforced my long-held belief that structural alignment is the biggest kept secret in health care. Every day I get to witness healing "miracles" as my team and I deliver on the promise of rebuilding bodies.

Chiropractors all over the world see "miracles" every week, if not every day, but the goal is for them to be consistent and predictable. The miracle isn't really the outcome that you're looking for. The outcome you're seeking is restoration of the natural conditions whereby your body can be healthy and operate at its peak potential. From that point, it's likely to have a much greater capacity to fix itself. Of course, alignment isn't the only thing that can go wrong. There can be, and often are, issues with one's nutritional and emotional health that play important roles. Those are both hugely important topics as well, and ones that we also address with our patients. Together, these three pillars—structure, nutrition, and emotions—form the triad of health. They influence each other and the ultimate goal for health-conscious people is to balance all three pillars to reach the rare air where true wellness exists.

There are all kinds of things you can do to improve your health. If you want to get fit, it's going to take several weeks or months before you start seeing the health benefits you want to see. If you want to start working on your emotional stress, that too will take some time—regardless of the approach you use—to rewire the way that your brain sees things. Getting your spine properly adjusted, on the other hand, creates a relatively instantaneous shift, and initiates a positive cascade effect through the whole body. From your heart to your brain to your digestive system, joints, and muscles, everything gets an upgrade from restored proper alignment and the release of physical stress. It's the fastest and most impactful way that I have found to upgrade health and performance, taking nothing away from the importance of good nutrition, exercise, and stress reduction, all of which should also be pursued.

I have revealed the absolutely necessary foundations of mastering the art and science of moving well. It all begins with an appreciation of the fact that your alignment matters, that it is inextricably linked to every function and system in your body, and that there is a predictable process by which it goes wrong.

The discovery that bones can misalign in directions from which your body cannot retrieve them is groundbreaking. Not only do we have the exact mechanism to explain body pain and posture problems for the first time, but we also understand how to reverse the process. Once you understand the foundational mechanisms by which something works, you have a much greater ability to control it. This is why ABC™ is changing the standard for structural healthcare the world over. It has solved the great problem that plagues most practitioners, which is that not everyone gets better from their methods. Not only that, you cannot accurately predict which patients will respond well and which will not. This is what happens when you address only the secondary compensation effect of the deeper cause. I unknowingly practiced that way for years, and it was only when I become a patient in real need myself that I began searching for the deepest underlying cause. This new methodology has made bigger strides towards predictable and consistent structural healthcare than any other healing art of which I am currently aware.

The knowledge of how and why a body becomes poorly aligned allows you to make much better choices in your daily life. For example, the unfortunate fact that most chairs are slowly destroying your body is inconvenient at best and highly annoying at worst. Yet, at the same time, it is a liberating truth of which to be aware because there is nothing more entrapping and disempowering than feeling like a victim. Not understanding the reason you keep experiencing pain, injuries, poor health, and plateaus in your physical performance is the worst case scenario because it leaves you waiting and hoping for change. Unless you do something about it, that change does not come, and this is why so many people experience a relapsing and remitting cycle of pain and dysfunction. The only way out of that particular karmic cul de sac is to tackle the root cause of the problem.

Seeing an ABC™ practitioner has the potential to unlock levels of health and performance about which you have long since forgotten. An interesting point to ponder is that you are not gaining anything new when you go through the unwinding journey, you are simply unveiling the inherent structure you've always had but unfortunately lost under layers of mechanical injuries. In this way, the process of structural correction is like stepping back in time. The farther down the healing path you go, the more function you will unlock, until eventually, you find yourself saying things like, "I feel better at thirty-six than I did at eighteen." That is how I feel about my own body now, which is remarkable considering the amount of traumatic physical stress I have put myself through over the years.

As an ABC™ practitioner, I hear these kinds of remarks all day long. Over time, the stories of years (or decades) of pain disappearing become commonplace, even expected. I never tire of hearing, however, are the stories of patients' lives and physical performance improving as a result of this methodology. People frequently report being able to run faster, hit a golf ball further, fly up the stairs, breathe more easily, wake up feeling rested, get to the end of the day without feeling wiped out, ski better this year than they ever have before, recover much faster from big workouts, feel more balanced when doing their sport, pick up their children without pain, get back to work after a long period off, look and feel more confident in their bodies, and better handle emotional stress. The list of improvements goes on and on, simply because you live life through your physical body. When you get your body back, you get your life back.

Experiences of improved function are the best sign of deep and significant progress in your structure. Pain has been, and will always be, a bit of a red herring. No one wants pain, but you can be completely pain-free and still drop tomorrow from a heart attack.

You can also live in a world of pain, yet have all of your test results come back negative for suspected issues. Therefore, health has been, and will always be, about regaining and maintaining the highest levels of function that you can.

A quick Google search will reveal your nearest ABC™ practitioner. If you cannot find one in your area, it is still worth enquiring with local chiropractic offices. Some chiropractic doctors practice it, but don't advertise that fact. Alternatively, you can travel for your treatment and still make enough progress to get the positive momentum you need and desire. At my centre in Hampton, London, we frequently welcome patients who fly from overseas to see us for brief periods of intensive care. More commonly, people drive anywhere from one and a half to five hours in one direction to get adjusted. It is certainly more inconvenient to travel, but if you want these sorts of results, it is necessary. In the UK, for example, no matter where you live, you are unlikely to be more than three to five hours from an ABC™ practitioner. Help is there if you need it.

The Standing Well, Sleeping Well, Sitting Well, and Moving Well chapters were written to help you master the physical forces on your body. Remember that gravity will show up, relentlessly, day-in and day-out. It is a reliable tormentor to skeletal frames. So you had better show up prepared, or errors in these habits will eventually contribute to long-term alignment problems and all of the undesirable consequences that come along with that. If you do nothing more than commit to mastering these areas of your lifestyle, you will significantly decrease the physical stress load on your body and halt the steady postural degeneration that is so common in our modern society. With a reduced stress load, there is always a greater capacity for healing. When your daily renewal habits meet or exceed the burden of daily stress, you will have mastered your health.

Thank you very much for reading. Live in alignment and thrive at life,

Richard

References

1. Cohen, RG, Vasavada, AN, Wesit MM, et al. Mobility and upright posture are associated with different aspects of cognition in older adults. Frontiers in aging neuroscience, DOI: 10.3389/fnagi.2016.00257.

2. Eric Jensen. "Moving With The Brain In Mind," Educational Leadership 58, no. 3 (2000):34-37

3. Lenon, J. Shealy, N. Cady, R. Et al. Posture and respiratory modulation of automatic function, pain and health. AJPM, 1994: 4:36-39

4. ptjournal.apta.org/content/early/2016/05/11/ptj.20150660

5. Gatchel RJ, Peng YB, Peters ML. The biopsychosocial approach to chronic pain: Scientific Advances and Future Directions. Psychological Bulletin, July 2007, DOI: 10.1037/0033-2909.133.4.581

6. Resnick, M. Postural changes due to fatigue. Computers and Industrial Engineering, 31 (1) (1996), pp. 491-494

7. nhs.uk/live-well/sleep-and-tiredness/eight-energy-stealers/

8. P.P. Reddy, T.P. Reddy, J. Roig-Francoli, L. Cone, B. Sivan, W.R. DeFoor, et al. The impact of the alexander technique on improving posture and surgical ergonomics during minimally invasive surgery: Pilot study Journal of Urology, 186 (2011), pp. 1658-1662

9. Zafar H, Albarrati A Alghadir AH et al. Effect of Different Head-Neck Postures on the Respiratory Function in Healthy Males. Biomed Res Int. 2018 Jul 12;2018:4518269.

10. Albarrati A, Zafar H, Alghadir AH et al. Effect of Upright and Slouched Sitting Postures on the Respiratory Muscle Strength in Healthy Young Males. Biomed Res Int. 2018 Feb 25;2018:3058970

11. Kocjan, J. Adamek M, Gzik-Zroska, B. Network of breathing. Multifunctional role of the diaphragm: a review. Adv Respir Med 2017;85(4):224-232

12. Dimitriadis, Z., Kapreli E., Strimpakos N, et al. Pulmonary Function of Patients with Chronic Neck Pain: A Spirometry Study. Respiratory Care April 2014, 59 (4) 543-549;

13. Schunemann, H. Grant, B. Trevisan, M. Pulmonary Function Is a Long-term Predictor of Mortality in the General Population. Chest 2000; 118:656-664).

14. Kado, D, MD et al: Hyperkyphotic Posture predicts Mortality In Older Community-Dwelling Men and Women: A Prospective Study, JAGS: 1662, Oct 2004

15. Kado DM, Huang MH, Barrett-Connor E, Greendale GA. Hyperkyphotic posture and poor physical functional ability in older community-dwelling men and women: the Rancho Bernardo study. J Gerontol A Biol Sci Med Sci. 2005;60(5):633–7.

16. Kado DM, Huang MH, Nguyen CB, Barrett-Connor E, Greendale GA. Hyperkyphotic posture and risk of injurious falls in older persons: the Rancho Bernardo Study. J Gerontol A Biol Sci Med Sci. 2007;62(6):652–7

17. Huang MH, Barrett-Connor E, Greendale GA, Kado DM. Hyperkyphotic posture and risk of future osteoporotic fractures: the Rancho Bernardo study. J Bone Miner Res. 2006;21(3):419–23.

18. Wannamethee, S., Shaper, A., Lennon, L. & Whincup, P. (2006) Height loss in older men: associations with total mortality and incidence of cardiovascular disease. Archives of Internal Medicine, 166 (22) 2546- 2552.

19. Gold. et al. Straight Back Syndrome: positive response to spinal manipulation and adjunctive therapy – A case report. J Can

Chiropr Assoc. 2013 Jun; 57(2): 143–149.

20. Datey KK, Deshmukh MM, Engineer SD, Dalvi CP. Straight back syndrome. Br Heart J. 1964;26:614–619.

21. Deuchars, J., Edwards, I. (2007). Bad posture could raise your blood pressure. Journal of Neuroscience 27(31):8324-8333.

22. Carnet, DR, Cuddey, AJ, yap AJ. Power posing: brief nonverbal displays affect neuroendocrine levels and risk tolerance. Psychol Science. 2010, Oct; 21(10): 1363-8.

23. Quentin F. Gronau, Sara Van Erp, Daniel W. Heck, et al. Comprehensive Results in Social Psychology. 2017;2(1):123–138

24. Arnette, SL. Pettijohn II, TF. The effects of posture on self-percieved leadership. International Journal Of Business and Social Science. 2012: Vol 3, No. 14.

25. Bohns V, Wiltermuth S., sciencedirect.com/science/article/pii/S0022103111001612 Journal of Experimental Social Psychology. 2012 Jan;48(1):341–345.

26. Brinol P, Petty R, Wagner B. Body posture affects self-evaluation: A self-validation approach. European Journal Of Psychology. (2009). 39, 1053-1064

27. Riskind JH. They stoop to conquer: Guiding and self-regulatory functions of physical posture after success and failure. Journal of personality and social psychology. 1984, Vol. 47, No. 3, 479-493.

28. J. Gergley. Latent Effect of Passive Static Stretching on Driver Clubhead Speed, Distance, Accuracy, and Consistent Ball Contact in Young Male Competitive Golfers. Journal of Strength and Conditioning Research: https://journals.lww.com/nsca-jscr/toc/2010/12000

29. Simic L, Sarabon N, Markovic G. Does pre-exercise static stretching inhibit maximal muscular performance? A meta-analytical review. https://www.ncbi.nlm.nih.gov/pubmed/22316148. 2013

Mar;23(2):131-48.

30. Kay, A., Blazevich, A. Effect of Acute Static Stretch on Maximal Muscle Performance: A Systematic Review. Med Sci Sports Exerc. 2012 Jan;44(1):154-64.

31. 3. Robbins, S, Waked, S. Hazard of deceptive advertising of athletic footwear" Br J Sports Med. 1997 Dec; 31(4): 299–303.

32. Christine D. Pollard, Justin A. Ter Har, J.J. Hannigan, Marc F. Norcross. "Influence of Maximal Running Shoes on Biomechanics Before and After a 5K Run". Orthopaedic Journal of Sports Medicine, 2018; 6 (6)

33. Rice H, Jamison S, Davis I. Footwear Matters: Influence of Footwear and Foot Strike on Load Rates during Running. Med Sci Sports Exerc. 2016 Dec;48(12):2462-2468.

34. "The Shocking 'Text Neck' X-Rays That Shows Children As Young As SEVEN Are Becoming Hunch Backs Because Of Their Addiction To Smart Phones" Daily Mail Australia, October 15, 2015, www.dailmail.co.uk/news/article-3274835/Shocking-X-rays-teenagers-text-neck.html

35. Ren, S. Et al. (2016). Effect of pillow height on the biomechanics of the head-neck complex: investigation of the cranio-cervical pressure and cervical spine alignment. PeerJ. 4: e2397.

36. James A. Levine. "Get Up! Why Your Chair Is Killing You And What You Can Do About It" (New York: St. Martin's Press, 2014)

37. J Lennert Veerman, Genevieve N. Healy, et al. "Television Viewing Time and Reduced Life Expectancy: A Life Table Analysis," British Journal Of Sports Medicine 46 (2012): 927-930

38. Mary Shaw, Richard Mitchell, Danny Dorling. "Time For A Smoke? One Cigarette Reduces Your Life by 11 Minutes," BMJ 320, no. 7226 (2000): 53.

39. Rice H, Jamison S, Davis I. Footwear Matters: Influence of Footwear and Foot Strike on Load Rates during Running. Med Sci

Sports Exerc. 2016 Dec;48(12):2462-2468.

40. "Health Topics: Physical Activity." World Health Organisation, www.who.int/topics/physical_activity/en/

41. Eric Jensen. "Moving With The Brain In Mind," Educational Leadership 58, no. 3 (2000):34-37

42. https://www.ukactive.com/events/inactive-brits-spend-twice-as-long-on-toilet-per-week-as-they-do-exercising/

43. Biwas, A, Ah, PI, Faulkner, GE, et al. "Sedentary time and its association with risk for disease incidence, mortality, and hospitalization in adults: a systematic review and meta-analysis." Ann Intern Med. 2015 Jan20;162(2):123-32

44. Brito, L, Ricardo, D, Soares de Araujo, D, et al. "Ability to Sit and Rise from the Floor as a Predictor of All-Cause Mortality" (2010) European Journal Of Preventive Cardiology.

45. James A. Levine. "Get Up! Why Your Chair Is Killing You And What You Can Do About It" (New York: St. Martin's Press, 2014)

About the Author

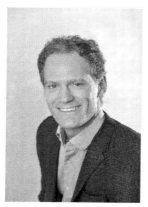

Dr. Richard Gliddon is a registered chiropractor and founder of the SpineCentral Structural Correction centre in London, UK. He is passionate about all things related to health and sports, and when he is not working with clients, he is training for and competing in triathlons, playing tennis, or practising calisthenics. He specialises in Advanced BioStructural Correction™, Applied Kinesiology, Neuro-Emotional Technique, and Lifestyle Wellness Solutions to help people naturally recover their peak health and performance.

www.spinecentral.co.uk

facebook.com/richardgliddonDC